Basic and Clinical
Pharmacology
made memorable

For Churchill Livingstone:

Publisher: Timothy Horne
Project Editor: Janice Urquhart
Copy Editor: Teresa Brady
Indexer: Hilary Flenley
Design Direction: Erik Bigland
Project Controller: Nancy Arnott
Page Layout: Kate Walshaw

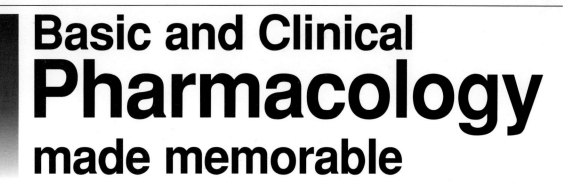

Basic and Clinical
Pharmacology
made memorable

Jason Luty BSc MB ChB
Research Assistant, Department of Pharmacology, Bristol University, Bristol, UK

Patrick Harrison BSc
Research Scientist, Department of Pharmacology, Bristol University, Bristol, UK

Illustrated by Robert Britton

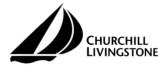

CHURCHILL
LIVINGSTONE

NEW YORK EDINBURGH LONDON MADRID MELBOURNE SAN FRANCISCO TOKYO 1997

CHURCHILL LIVINGSTONE
Medical Division of Pearson Professional Limited

Distributed in the United States of America by
Churchill Livingstone Inc., 650 Avenue of the Americas,
New York, N.Y. 10011, and by associated companies,
branches and representatives throughout the world.

First published 1997

ISBN 0 443 05598 X

British Library Cataloguing in Publication Data
A catalogue record for this book is available from the
British Library

Library of Congress Cataloging in Publication Data
A catalog record for this book is available from the
Library of Congress

Medical knowledge is constantly changing. As new
information becomes available, changes in treatment,
procedures, equipment and the use of drugs become
necessary. The author and the publishers have, as
far as it is possible, taken care to ensure that the
information given in the text is accurate and up to
date. However, readers are strongly advised to
confirm that the information, especially with regard
to drug usage, complies with current legislation and
standards of practice.

The
publisher's
policy is to use
**paper manufactured
from sustainable forests**

Produced by Longman Asia Ltd, Hong Kong
NPCC/01

Preface

Basic and Clinical Pharmacology will be of interest to any member of the biomedical professions, including students of medicine, nursing, dentistry, pharmacology and pharmacy. The book has been written primarily for medical students preparing for their second MB pharmacology exams.

Although there are several excellent textbooks which are suitable for full-time students of pharmacology, these are often too detailed and cumbersome for the requirements of medical students. Furthermore, many pharmacology textbooks include older, obsolete agents and details regarding the chemical structure and classification of drugs which are not clinically useful. Hence we have only used the most widely prescribed agents to illustrate the basic principles of pharmacology. This minimises the number of drugs named in the main text, and will reduce the burden placed on medical students who are also required to contend with anatomy, biochemistry and physiology.

Jason Luty is a research assistant in the Department of Pharmacology at Bristol University. He is a qualified clinician with practical experience of anaesthesia, psychiatry, cardiology and neurology.

Patrick Harrison is a research scientist in the Department of Pharmacology at Bristol University. He is presently using techniques of molecular pharmacology to investigate the action of alcohol on the differentiation of cultured cells.

Bristol

J.L.
P.H.

Acknowledgements

The authors gratefully acknowledge
the assistance of Dr Eamonn Kelly,
Mr Stuart Mundell, Miss Penny Nelmes,
Dr Alastair Poole, Dr Christopher Lote,
Mr Jerry Jaymayne, Dr Caroline Brown,
Mr Christopher Mahon, Dr Sarah Utting,
Dr and Mrs Naeem Malik, Dr Geoff Dalton,
Dr Tassem Chowdry, Dr Leyla Sania and
Dr Catherine Dukes.

Contents

GABA Hey .

1

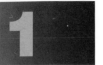

How drugs work: receptors

A drug is a chemical compound which is administered to produce a desirable physiological or psychological effect. All drug molecules interact with biological structures such as protein receptors and enzymes. This interaction triggers a series of steps that ultimately results in a physiological change which constitutes the drug's effect. Side-effects are the undesirable changes which are also produced by a drug. All drugs produce side-effects because drugs produce multiple physiological effects.

Drug receptors are molecules which bind drugs and initiate a response. There are several types of drug receptors and mechanisms of action.

1. Neurohumoral receptors: Neurohumoral receptors are macromolecules which bind drugs, hormones or neurotransmitters and initiate a cellular response. In pharmacology, neurohumoral receptors are often called merely 'receptors' although many drugs act at sites other than neurohumoral receptors. *Receptor occupancy* is the proportion of receptors physically bound to a drug at any instant.

An agonist is a drug that binds to a receptor and produces a cellular response. An antagonist is a drug that prevents the actions of an agonist. Some antagonists interact with a receptor but can be displaced by another drug. These are known as competitive antagonists because they compete with other drugs to interact with the receptor. The effects of other antagonists cannot be overcome by adding an excess of agonist.

These are known as noncompetitive or irreversible antagonists. Noncompetitive antagonists may interact with a receptor and form a permanent attachment to it thereby preventing any other drug from acting on that receptor. Alternatively they may prevent an agonist acting by interfering with a component of the cellular response other than at the receptor site.

2. Enzyme inhibitors: Many drugs act by inhibiting particular enzymes. The action of reversible enzyme inhibitors may be overcome by adding an excess of substrate. The action of irreversible enzyme inhibitors cannot be overcome by additional substrate. Drugs usually act as reversible enzyme inhibitors. Notice that the action of enzymes is blocked by *inhibitors* whereas the action of agonists at neurohumoral receptors is blocked by *antagonists*.

3. Drugs acting on ion channels: There are two kinds of ion channels: voltage-operated ion channels (VOCs) which open in response to a change in the electrical potential across them, and receptor-operated ion channels (ROCs) which open in response to an agonist (such as a neurotransmitter). Drugs can block or enhance the conduction of ions through channels.

4. Other mechanisms: Drugs may exert their action by modifying DNA replication or synthesis of protein. Alternatively they may block the storage, release or reuptake of neurotransmitters or their precursors.

Examples of different mechanisms of drug action

Receptor type	Example	Mode of action	Use
Neurohumoral receptors			
Agonist	Salbutamol	Agonist at β_2-adrenergic receptors	Asthma
Competitive antagonist	Atropine	Competitive antagonist at muscarinic receptors	Bradycardia (heart rate less than 60 beats per minute)
Noncompetitive antagonist	Phenoxybenzamine	Noncompetitive antagonist at α-adrenoceptors	Antihypertensive (rarely used)
Enzyme inhibitors			
Reversible	Enalapril	Reversible inhibitor of angiotensin-converting enzyme. (Prevents angiotensin II synthesis)	Antihypertensive
Irreversible	Aspirin	Irreversible inhibitor of the enzyme cyclooxygenase. (Prevents eicosanoid synthesis)	Analgesic (pain killer)
Ion channel			
Blocker	Nifedipine	Blocks voltage-operated calcium channels	Antihypertensive
Facilitator	Diazepam	Enhances chloride flux at gamma aminobutyric acid A (GABA$_A$) receptor	Sedative (used to relieve anxiety or insomnia)
Inhibition of DNA replication	Cyclophosphamide	Cross-links DNA and inhibits DNA replication	Cytotoxic (used in cancer treatment)
Inhibition of protein synthesis	Erythromycin	Inhibits bacterial protein synthesis	Antibiotic

How drugs work

- A drug is a chemical compound which is administered to produce a desirable physiological or psychological effect

- Drug receptors are molecules which bind drugs and initiate a response

- There are several types of receptor such as neurohumoral receptors (which normally respond to endogenous hormones or neurotransmitters), enzymes, ion channels and DNA

- An agonist is a drug which binds to a (neurohumoral) receptor and produces a cellular response

- An antagonist is any drug which prevents the action of an agonist

- The effect of a competitive antagonist can be overcome by using an excess of an agonist

- The effects of a noncompetitive antagonist cannot be overcome by additional agonist

- The action of a reversible enzyme inhibitor may be overcome by adding an excess of substrate

- The action of irreversible enzyme inhibitors cannot be overcome by additional substrate

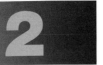

Signal transduction:
G-proteins and second messengers

Cellular responses include contraction of muscle cells, conduction of action potentials and secretion of neurotransmitters. Signal transduction is the mechanism by which a cellular response is initiated after an agonist binds to a receptor. This may involve activation of ion channels and changes in gene expression. However a common sequence of events involves activation of a G-protein, synthesis of a second messenger and a subsequent phosphorylation cascade which activates (or inhibits) intracellular enzymes.

G-proteins

G-proteins (guanine nucleotide-binding proteins) consist of three subunits (α-, β- and γ-subunits) which associate with membrane-bound receptors in the inactive state. The α-subunit binds a guanosine diphosphate (GDP) molecule in this state. When an agonist binds to the receptor, a conformational change occurs causing the α-subunit to release the GDP molecule and bind guanosine triphosphate (GTP). The α- and $\beta\gamma$-subunits then dissociate from the receptor and go on to produce a range of effects including activation enzymes or inhibition of ion channels (see later). Gradually the α-subunit degrades GTP to GDP whereupon the α-subunit will recombine with free $\beta\gamma$-subunits and a receptor. The whole receptor–G-protein complex will then remain inactive until another agonist molecule binds to the receptor. There are many different types of α-, β- and γ-subunits which produce different effects.

Second-messenger systems

Second messengers are mobile intracellular molecules which form part of the transduction system. Examples of these include cyclic adenosine monophosphate (cAMP), diacylglycerol (DAG), inositol trisphosphate (IP_3) and calcium ions. cAMP is synthesised by adenylyl cyclase after activation by the free α-subunit of a specific G-protein, Gs. cAMP can activate protein kinase A (PKA). A single activated PKA molecule may phosphorylate several other enzyme molecules which may be of different types. This produces a 'cascade' in which one type of kinase enzyme phosphorylates and may activate several others. This cascade amplifies the signal and can ultimately activate many different response pathways. The α-subunits of the Gi class of G-proteins inhibit adenylyl cyclase.

Phospholipase C (PLC) activation may occur in response to the free α-subunits of the specific G-proteins, Gq or G11. This enzyme breaks down the membrane phospholipid, phosphatidyl-inositol-4,5-bisphosphate (PIP_2), to produce two second messengers, diacylglycerol (DAG) and inositol-1,4,5-trisphosphate (IP_3). The DAG activates protein kinase C (PKC) which phosphorylates other enzymes, thereby initiating a cascade. IP_3 stimulates release of calcium from intracellular stores. This rise in intracellular calcium directly activates some forms of PKC or binds calmodulin in order to activate other enzymes and produce cellular responses.

Other secondary messengers include cyclic guanosine monophosphate (cGMP) which probably activates cGMP-dependent protein kinase (PKG).

Intracellular phosphoprotein phosphatases can dephosphorylate proteins and thereby terminate the effects of phosphorylation cascades.

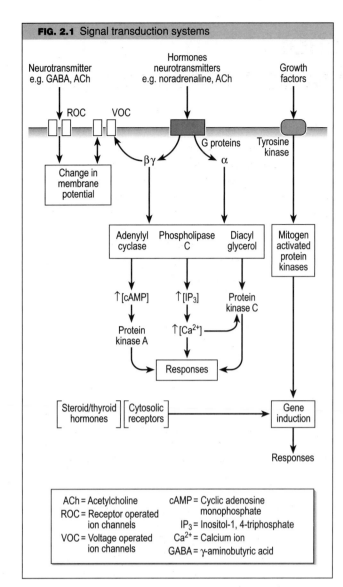

FIG. 2.1 Signal transduction systems

ACh = Acetylcholine
ROC = Receptor operated ion channels
VOC = Voltage operated ion channels
cAMP = Cyclic adenosine monophosphate
IP_3 = Inositol-1, 4-triphosphate
Ca^{2+} = Calcium ion
GABA = γ-aminobutyric acid

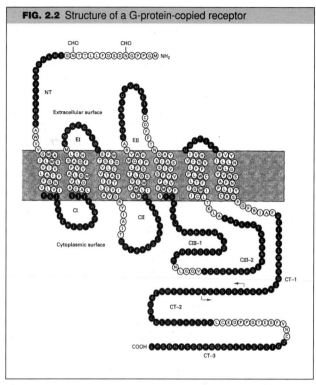

FIG. 2.2 Structure of a G-protein-copied receptor

G-proteins and second messengers

- Signal transduction is the mechanism by which a cellular response is initiated after an agonist binds to a receptor

- One signal transduction system involves activation of a G-protein, synthesis of a second messenger and a subsequent phosphorylation cascade which activates (or inhibits) intracellular enzymes

- G-proteins (guanine nucleotide-binding proteins) consist of three different subunits (α, β and γ). These dissociate from membrane-bound receptors following binding of an agonist and may then activate effector systems

- Dissociation of the subunits occurs following binding of GTP to the α-subunit. This is gradually hydrolysed to GDP which then allows reassociation of the G-protein subunits with the receptor. This terminates their action

- Second messengers are mobile intracellular molecules which form part of the transduction system

- Cyclic adenosine monophosphate (cAMP) is one second messenger. It is synthesised by adenylyl cyclase following activation by G-proteins

- cAMP activates protein kinase A which phosphorylates many different intracellular enzymes. This produces a phosphorylation cascade which activates or inhibits other enzymes to produce a cellular response

- Diacylglycerol and inositol-1,4,5-trisphosphate (IP_3) are also second messengers. They activate protein kinase C and stimulate release of calcium from intracellular stores to produce cellular responses

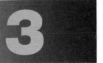

Other signal transduction systems

Receptor-operated
ion channels (ROCs)

These ion channels open in response to binding of an agonist such as acetylcholine at nicotinic receptors. ROCs may cause cellular depolarisation or hyperpolarisation which subsequently modulates voltage-operated ion channels (VOCs). This may initiate chains of action potentials. ROCs and VOCs also allow calcium influx causing activation of the calcium/calmodulin pathway and other responses (including neurotransmitter release). (See the table for examples of ROCs.) VOCs may also be modulated by a direct interaction with the βγ-subunits of some G-proteins.

The tyrosine and
MAP–kinase pathway

Receptors for insulin and some growth hormones express a tyrosine kinase enzyme which, upon activation, initiates a signalling pathway by phosphorylation and activation of certain mitogen-activated proteins (MAPs). This kinase phosphorylates specific tyrosine residues in other proteins, whereas the other kinases involved in signal transduction usually phosphorylate serine or threonine amino acid residues. This MAP–kinase pathway ultimately leads to changes in gene expression, cell growth and differentiation.

The NO system

Nitric oxide (NO) is released from endothelial cells to relax vascular smooth muscle and produce vasodilation. Some vasodilator drugs act via this system. NO is synthesised intracellularly from arginine by the enzyme nitric oxide synthase (also known as NADPH diaphorase). The NO then diffuses into other cells and directly activates guanylate cyclase to produce the secondary messenger cyclic

guanosine monophosphate (cGMP). This may activate protein kinase G and other effector systems to produce a cellular response. NO has a short half-life (~5 seconds) therefore it only has a local action. NO may act as a neurotransmitter and it is a toxic product released by immune cells.

Steroid–thyroid hormone receptors

Steroid and thyroid hormones bind to intracellular receptors which are normally located within the nucleus. The hormone–receptor complex can then bind directly to specific sites on DNA to alter gene expression, leading to changes in cell growth and differentiation.

Arachidonic acid cascade

Arachidonic acid is formed from membrane phospholipids by activation of the enzyme phospholipase A_2. It may also have signal functions of its own. However, arachidonic acid is also converted into eicosanoids (prostaglandins and leukotrienes) by the enzyme cyclooxygenase. These are important inflammatory mediators. Many drugs inhibit this pathway. For example glucocorticoids produce downregulation of cyclooxygenase, whilst nonsteroidal antiinflammatory drugs, such as aspirin, inhibit this enzyme.

The time course of
transduction systems

Responses involving ROCs are rapid and occur over a timescale of a few milliseconds. Responses involving G-protein-linked receptors are slower and develop over a few seconds. Responses to steroid–thyroid hormones and growth factors involve changes in gene expression and protein synthesis. These responses take several hours or days.

Examples of receptor-operated ion channels (ROCs)

Receptor	Agonist	Ion channel	Effect	Location
Nicotinic Cholinergic	Acetylcholine	$Na^+/K^+/Ca^{2+}$ (cations)	Depolarisation	Neuromuscular junction Autonomic ganglia CNS
Ionotropic excitatory amino acid receptors	Glutamate	$Na^+/K^+/Ca^{2+}$ (cations)	Depolarisation	CNS
GABA$_A$	GABA (γ-aminobutyric acid)	Cl^-	Hyperpolarisation	Brain
Glycine	Glycine	Cl^-	Hyperpolarisation	Spinal cord

FIG. 3.1 Other signal transduction systems

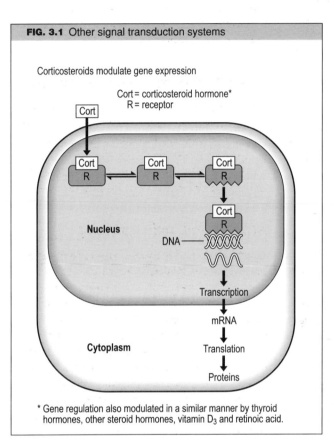

Corticosteroids modulate gene expression

Cort = corticosteroid hormone*
R = receptor

Nucleus

DNA

Transcription

mRNA

Cytoplasm

Translation

Proteins

* Gene regulation also modulated in a similar manner by thyroid hormones, other steroid hormones, vitamin D$_3$ and retinoic acid.

FIG. 3.2 Model of a receptor-operated channel, e.g. nicotinic receptor

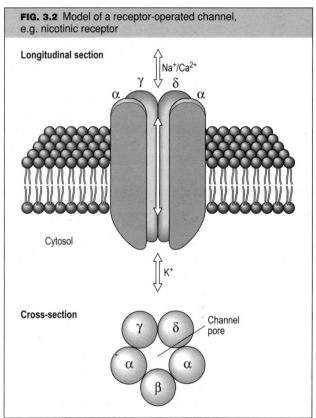

Longitudinal section

Na^+/Ca^{2+}

Cytosol

K^+

Cross-section

Channel pore

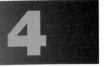

Drug receptor theory: concentration–response curves

The ability of an agonist to produce a response depends on affinity and efficacy. The *affinity* of a drug is an estimate of the force of attraction between the drug and a receptor. The *efficacy* is the capacity of a drug to activate a receptor once it has bound.

As a tissue is exposed to increasing concentrations of drug, progressively more receptors are activated and the observed response increases. However, there is a maximal response, after which an increase in concentration has no further effect. A concentration–response curve shows the response produced by different concentrations (or doses) of a drug (Fig. 4.1a). These curves approximate to rectangular hyperbolas.

Drugs produce responses over a wide range of concentrations. Consequently, concentration–response curves are usually transformed into log concentration–response curves by calculating the logarithm of the concentration (Fig 4.1b). These approximate to sigmoid curves.

Most full agonists need only to occupy a fraction of the available receptors on a cell to produce a maximal response. The cell (or tissue) is then said to have *spare receptors*.

The molar concentration of agonist required to produce a half-maximal response is called the *EC50*. This is an estimate of potency. A full agonist with a low potency will produce a log concentration–response curve which is parallel but to the right of a curve for a more potent full agonist (Fig. 4.1c).

The number of receptors on a cell is finite and some agonists have such a low efficacy that they cannot produce a maximal response even when all the available receptors are occupied. These drugs are called *partial agonists*. A log concentration–response curve for a partial agonist will exhibit a lower maximal response than the log concentration–response curve for a full agonist acting on the same receptors (Fig. 4.1d).

Antagonism

Competitive antagonists bind reversibly to receptors. They will compete with agonists for the available receptors. Hence, in the presence of a competitive antagonist, a higher concentration of agonist is needed to produce the same response (the extra agonist molecules may be considered to be displacing the antagonist from the receptors). A competitive antagonist will shift the log concentration–response for an agonist curve to the right (Fig. 4.1c). The pA_2 value is an estimate of antagonist potency. It is the logarithm of the concentration of antagonist that makes it necessary to double the concentration of agonist needed to elicit the original (submaximal) response.

Noncompetitive antagonists effectively block receptors permanently. They cannot be displaced from the receptors by increasing the concentration of an agonist. Under some conditions, there will be too few functional receptors remaining to produce the maximal response even if they are all occupied by full agonists. Hence a noncompetitive antagonist can reduce the maximal response of an agonist log concentration–response curve (Fig. 4.1d).

Positive cooperativity exists if the binding of one molecule of a drug increases the affinity of the receptor for a second molecule (some receptors need to bind more than one molecule to be activated). This will steepen the concentration–response curve. Similarly, *negative cooperativity* exists if binding of one drug molecule inhibits the binding of a second. This will flatten the concentration–response curve (Fig. 4.1e).

FIG. 4.1a–e Drug receptor theory

1a A typical dose response curve

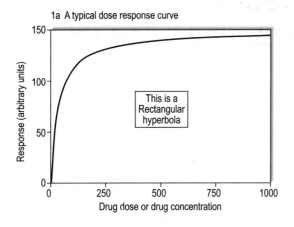

This is a Rectangular hyperbola

1b A typical log-dose response curve

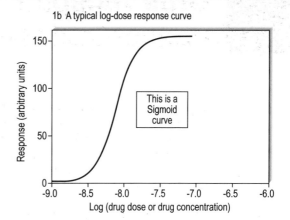

This is a Sigmoid curve

1c Log-dose response curves

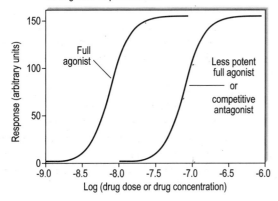

Full agonist

Less potent full agonist or competitive antagonist

1d Log-dose response curves

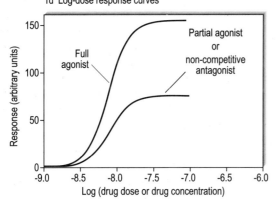

Full agonist

Partial agonist or non-competitive antagonist

1e Log-dose response curve to show cooperativity

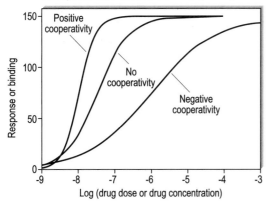

Positive cooperativity

No cooperativity

Negative cooperativity

5

Pharmacokinetics 1

Pharmacokinetics describes what happens to the drug once it has been administered. All drugs are absorbed, distributed and then excreted by the body.

Absorption

In order for most drugs to achieve their desired effect they must cross at least one membrane. The ability to cross a membrane will depend on several factors: the size and shape of the molecules of the drug, the lipid solubility and the ionic charge. Absorption is more efficient for small, lipid-soluble, electrically neutral molecules which can cross membranes easily.

Many drugs are either bases or acids and so the ionic charge will depend on the surrounding pH. Thus in the stomach acidic drugs will be more likely to be neutral, whilst basic drugs are more likely to be charged. The pK_a value is the pH where 50% of the drug is in the ionised form, and is derived from the Henderson–Hasselbach equation. For a base:

$$pK_a = pH + \log [BH^+]/[B]$$

For an acid:

$$pK_a = pH + \log [AH]/[A^-]$$

BH^+ = concentration of base in the
       ionised form
B = concentration of base in the
       un-ionised form
AH = concentration of acid in the
       un-ionised form
A^- = concentration of acid in the
       ionised form

These equations allow determination of the proportion of a base (e.g. pethidine) or acid (e.g. aspirin) that will be in the ionised form. Drugs in the un-ionised form will be absorbed more rapidly.

A drug may be administered by various routes, e.g. oral, injection (intravenous, intramuscular, subcutaneous), inhalation, topical, sublingual and rectal.

Drugs taken orally are absorbed in the gastrointestinal tract where they enter the portal circulation. Some drugs can alter absorption in the gastrointestinal tract by affecting motility, pH or gastric emptying

(e.g. morphine). Many other factors such as systemic or gastrointestinal diseases, pain, the presence of food or pregnancy will alter absorption. Before entering the systemic circulation, these drugs are passed through the liver, where they may be metabolised by enzymes. This metabolism of drugs is known as the *first-pass effect*. *Prodrugs* are initially inert; when metabolised they become active. Codeine is a prodrug.

Rectal and sublingual drugs are absorbed directly into the systemic circulation and avoid this effect. Drugs administered topically are only absorbed into the circulation if they are sufficently lipophilic. Intravenous injection introduces a drug directly into the circulation, whilst intramuscular and subcutaneous injections produce a slower absorption into the circulation.

Distribution

Drugs are not evenly distributed throughout the body. Highly lipid-soluble drugs, such as thiopentone, are initially distributed in the brain and are then redistributed throughout the body. The redistribution of thiopentone following intravenous injection terminates its action as an anaesthetic.

The volume through which a drug is distributed is termed the *volume of distribution* (V_d). There are three main compartments through which a drug may be distributed: the vascular compartment (i.e. the bloodstream), ≈5% of body weight; the extracellular compartment, ≈15% of body weight, and the intracellular compartment, ≈30% of body weight. Drugs having large molecules and those which bind highly to plasma proteins remain in the vascular compartment; drugs which have a low lipid solubility are distributed in the vascular compartment and the extracellular fluid, whilst lipid-soluble drugs are distributed through the three compartments.

The volume of distribution can be calculated from the following equation:

$$V_d = Q/C_p$$

where V_d is the volume of distribution
Q is the total amount of drug
C_p is the concentration of the drug in the plasma.

FIG. 5.1 The relationship between plasma concentration and time for most drugs

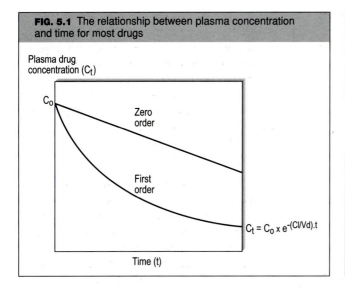

Plasma drug concentration (C_t)

C_0

Zero order

First order

$C_t = C_0 \times e^{-(Cl/Vd).t}$

Time (t)

Prescribing in the elderly

Elderly people are more sensitive to the side-effects of drugs (particularly sedation, constipation and electrolyte imbalances) and they often have impaired abilities to metabolise and excrete drugs. Hence many drugs are given at reduced doses in the elderly often using half the dose of a healthy adult.

Phase I and II metabolism

Drug metabolism involves two kinds of biochemical reaction. Phase I reactions introduce a relatively reactive group, such as a hydroxyl, by oxidation, hydroxylation, dealkylation or deamination. These functional groups are then conjugated with larger substituents such as glucuronyl, sulphate or acetyl groups in a Phase II reaction. These reactions normally decrease both the pharmacological activity and lipid solubility of a drug thereby inactivating the agent and increasing the rate of renal elimination.

Routes of drug administration

Route: example	Advantages	Disadvantages
Oral: aspirin	Cheap, convenient	First-pass effect. Drugs must be stable and be absorbed from the gut
Inhalation: salbutamol, halothane	Rapid entry into the bloodstream, direct access for bronchodilating drugs to the lungs	Only suitable for volatile drugs or those acting on airways
Sublingual: glyceryl trinitrate	Rapid entry avoiding the first-pass effect	Not all drugs can be absorbed this way
Injection Subcutaneous: insulin Intravenous: thiopentone Intramuscular: haloperidol	Rapid administration, avoids first pass	Inconvenient; intravenous occurs only in hospitals
Regional anaesthesia (e.g. epidural): lignocaine*	Avoids need for general anaesthesia	Technically difficult
Topical: corticosteroids	Minimises systemic side-effects	Site of action must be accessible, e.g. skin, joints
Rectal: diclofenac	Useful in patient unable to take drugs by mouth, i.e. due to vomiting	Absorption is unreliable

* See Ch. 32, Local anaesthetics

Pharmacokinetics 2

6

Elimination

In order to inactivate a drug, the body will either excrete the drug or its metabolites (removing it from the body normally via the kidney), and/or metabolise it (breaking the drug down). The metabolism of a drug can occur in different places in the body such as the liver, kidney or stomach wall. Drugs can cause an increased expression of metabolising enzymes, e.g. ethanol causes an increase of alcohol dehydrogenase in the stomach wall, and antiepileptic drugs cause an increase of cytochrome P450 in the liver. Metabolism of a drug can sometimes lead to pharmacologically active metabolites, e.g. benzodiazepines.

The concentration of a drug in the plasma will normally follow *first-order kinetics*, decreasing in a exponential manner. However, a few drugs, such as ethanol and phenytoin, have *zero-order kinetics*, and their concentration decreases in a linear fashion, particularly when the mechanism of elimination becomes overloaded or saturated.

The equation below states the relationship between plasma concentration and time.

$$C_t = C_0 \times e^{-(Cl/V_d)t}$$

where C_t is the concentration of the drug in the plasma at the time t
C_o is the initial plasma concentration of the drug
Cl is the clearance of the drug
V_d is the volume of distribution
t is a point in time.

Clearance is a way of describing the rate at which the body is eliminating the drug and is described by the following equation:

$$Cl = 0.69 \times V_d/(t_{\frac{1}{2}})$$

where Cl is the volume of plasma completely cleared of drug per unit of time
V_d is the volume of distribution
$t_{\frac{1}{2}}$ is the half-life of the drug.

If the rate of clearance is known, then it is possible to calculate the concentration of drug in the plasma by infusing new quantities of drug at the same rate as it is being eliminated. This is termed the *steady-state* plasma concentration.

$$C_{ss} = \text{infusion rate}/\text{clearance}$$

where C_{ss} is the steady-state plasma concentration.

When tablets are administered, the concentration in the plasma will fluctuate. It is possible to calculate the 'average' steady-state concentration (C_{av}) of the drug.

$$C_{av} = (\text{dose} \times F)/(\text{dosing interval} \times Cl)$$

where F is the bioavailability of the drug when administered orally and the dosing interval is the time between administration of doses.

The bioavailability is the proportion of drug which enters the systemic circulation. This takes into account any drug metabolism. (It should be noted that many pharmacokinetic parameters vary greatly between patients and even for a single patient on different occasions.) Bioavailability is defined by (see graph):

$$\frac{\text{area under the curve (when taken orally)}}{\text{area under the curve (when taken by intravenous injection)}}$$

The above equations use a single kinetic compartment model, i.e. they assume a drug is distributed evenly through a single compartment. Drugs such as thiopentone which undergo rapid redistribution from a central compartment require the use of a two-compartment pharmacokinetic model.

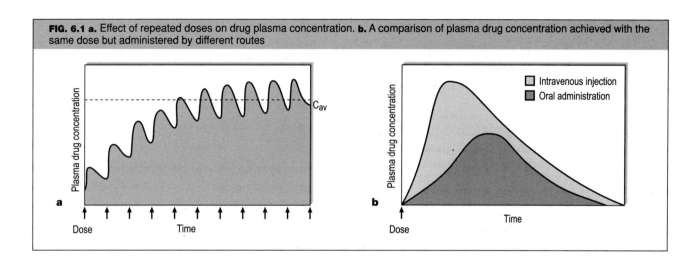

FIG. 6.1 a. Effect of repeated doses on drug plasma concentration. **b.** A comparison of plasma drug concentration achieved with the same dose but administered by different routes

REVISION AID

Pharmacokinetics

- Drugs are absorbed, distributed and then excreted by the body

- Important factors in determining membrane permeability include size, charge and lipophilicity

- The surrounding environment (pH) may influence the charge of a drug molecule, the proportion of drug in an uncharged/charged state can be determined from the Henderson–Hasselbach equation

- Many drugs pass through the liver before entering the systemic circulation, consequently they are subject to the *first pass effect*

- The distribution of a drug through the body will be determined by several factors, including size, charge and lipid solubility

- Most drugs are metabolised following *first-order kinetics* a few (e.g. ethanol) follow *zero-order kinetics*

- Clearance is a measure of the rate of elimination of a drug from the body

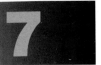

Voltage-operated
ion channels (VOCs)

Ion channels

The cell membrane actively exchanges ions, normally pumping Na^+, Ca^{2+} and Cl^- out and K^+ in. The table, 'The ion distribution in mammalian skeletal muscle', shows that excitable cells (such as nerve and muscle) have high concentrations of potassium inside and high concentrations of sodium and calcium outside. Hence there is a tendency for potassium to move out of cells (causing hyperpolarisation) and sodium and calcium ions to move in (causing depolarisation). These ionic movements occur by diffusion, down *chemical gradients* from regions of high concentration to regions of lower concentration.

Receptor-operated ion channels (ROCs) open in response to the binding of an agonist (such as acetylcholine or a secondary messenger) to a receptor site. Voltage-operated ion channels (VOCs) open or close in response to changes in the membrane potential. (The membrane potential is the difference in electrical charge between the outside and inside of the cell.) Some VOCs exhibit a preference for the conduction of a particular ion (especially voltage-operated calcium channels).

Ion channels are multisubunit proteins which span the cell membrane and contain a pore through which simple ions may flow. When a VOC opens there is a net flow of ions (such as Na^+, K^+, Ca^{2+} and Cl^-) through their respective channels down their *chemical* gradient. This produces an opposing *electrical* gradient which prevents further redistribution. The flow of ions through a VOC may be terminated by this opposing electrical gradient or by closing of the ion channel either spontaneously or in response to a change in the membrane potential. The flow of ions across the cell membrane alters the membrane potential.

Calcium entry through VOCs can produce cellular responses including neurotransmitter release or muscle contraction.

Many VOCs are thought to exist in three states: open (when they conduct ions); closed (when they do not conduct ions but may become open by an activating stimulus such as a depolarisation), and inactive (when they cannot conduct ions and will not open even in response to an activating stimulus).

Drugs acting on VOCs: calcium antagonists and local anaesthetics

Therapeutic drugs usually block VOCs. They may do this by physically blocking the ion channel or by altering the *channel kinetics*. This means that the channel may remain open for a shorter time, or it may open less frequently, or it may allow fewer ions to flow through it in a given time.

Some drugs, particularly those that modify receptor-operated ion channels, alter channel kinetics to enhance ion fluxes.

Local anaesthetic drugs, such as lignocaine, block voltage-operated sodium channels. Agents with a similar mechanism of action are used to treat epilepsy and cardiac arrhythmias. Local anaesthetics have a use-dependent action (the depth of block increases with use). This is partly because they block voltage-operated sodium channels at sites within the ion channel pore. Hence they can gain access to the channel more readily when it is open. Additionally they have a greater affinity for inactive channels which are more common in active membranes.

There are three main types of voltage-operated calcium channel (see the table 'Calcium channel subtypes'). Calcium antagonists, such as nifedipine and verapamil, used to treat hypertension and cardiac arrhythmias, block L-type voltage-operated calcium channels. Nifedipine acts by altering the channel kinetics, while verapamil acts by entering the channel and blocking it. This action of verapamil demonstrates use-dependence.

The ion distribution in mammalian skeletal muscle

Ion	Extracellular fluid, mM	Intracellular fluid	Equilibrium potential, mV
Na+	145	12 mM	+67
K+	4	155 mM	−98
Ca²⁺	1.5	0.1 μM	+129
Cl⁻	123	4.2 mM	−90

Calcium channel subtypes

Ca²⁺ channel type	Notes
L type	Voltage-activated. Large conductance. Long-lasting current. Found in heart and smooth muscle. Verapamil acts mainly on the heart, nifedipine on the smooth muscle. Verapamil clinically used for antidysrhythmia
N type	Voltage-activated. Moderate conductance. Moderately lasting current. Found on neurons. Important for neurotransmitter release. ω-Conotoxins will block. No clinical use
T type	Voltage-activated. Small conductance. Long-lasting current. Found throughout the body. Important for sinoatrial pacemaker. Octanol will block. No clinical use
P, Q, R types	Not much known

Action potentials

At the resting membrane potential (−60 mv), some potassium channels are open. However the electrical and chemical forces are equal, and there is no net movement of potassium ions across the membrane. If a cell becomes depolarised (more positively charged), potassium channels close and voltage-operated sodium channels open. Sodium ions flow into the cell and it becomes even more depolarised (the membrane potential moves towards the equilibrium potential for sodium).

Voltage-operated sodium channels close spontaneously after a few milliseconds and the membrane begins to repolarise (it becomes more negatively charged) as ions redistribute within the cell. This repolarisation activates voltage-operated potassium channels which help to further repolarise the cell until the resting membrane potential is restored.

This brief depolarisation is called an action potential. These can be conducted for long distances along the membranes of axons. They initiate the contraction of muscle cells and the release of neurotransmitters at neural synapses. Action potentials are initiated by depolarisation, typically by receptor-operated cation channels on postsynaptic membranes.

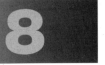

Acetylcholine

Biochemistry: Acetylcholine (ACh) is synthesised in cholinergic nerve terminals by the enzyme choline acetyltransferase, which adds an acetyl group (donated by coenzyme A) to choline. Choline is taken up by cells via a specific uptake system. ACh is broken down by the enzyme acetylcholinesterase (AChE) into choline and acetate. AChE is normally localised adjacent to the ACh receptor, allowing rapid breakdown of ACh. This is the mechanism by which the action of ACh is terminated. AChE can be competitively inhibited by neostigmine. Any ACh in the plasma is broken down by a different enzyme, butyrylcholinesterase (also known as pseudocholinesterase).

ACh is commonly stored in vesicles along with adenosine 5'-triphosphate (ATP) and peptides such as substance P or vasoactive intestinal peptide (VIP); these peptides are themselves neurotransmitters.

ACh receptors and their distribution:
There are two broad types of acetylcholine receptor: *muscarinic* receptors are activated by muscarine and are G-protein-linked receptors; the *nicotinic* receptors are activated by nicotine and are receptor-operated cation channels. Acetylcholine is a more potent agonist at muscarinic receptors than at nicotinic receptors.

There are known at present to be five types of muscarinic receptor; M_1, M_3 and M_5 couple to Gq/11, whilst M_2 and M_4 both couple to Gi/o. The drug atropine is a competitive antagonist of these receptors. The nicotinic receptors, like other cation channels, are made up of five subunits. There are five types of subunit; α, β, γ, δ and ϵ. Each subunit itself has different variations so the number of possible combinations is enormous. These different combinations have distinct pharmacological differences and distinct distributions. For instance, the muscle-type nicotinic receptor

is distinct from the nicotinic receptor in the CNS and also from the ganglionic type. Two molecules of ACh are required to activate a nicotinic receptor in skeletal muscle.

Curare is a competitive antagonist of these receptors.

ACh is found in the forebrain, midbrain and brainstem. Short cholinergic interneurons are found in the nucleus accumbens and striatum.

ACh is the neurotransmitter released from preganglionic neurons at the ganglia of the autonomic nervous system, in both sympathetic and parasympathetic branches. It acts on nicotinic receptors on the postganglionic neurons. It is also the transmitter released by postganglionic fibres of the parasympathetic system where it acts on muscarinic receptors. (ACh is released from postganglionic neurons of the sympathetic system, acting on muscarinic receptors to stimulate sweat glands. However, noradrenaline is the principal postganglionic neurotransmitter of the sympathetic nervous system.) Activation of muscarinic receptors by parasympathetic release of ACh causes a decreased rate and force of contractions; muscarinic antagonists such as atropine, have the opposite effect.

ACh is also the primary transmitter in the somatic efferent system where it stimulates nicotinic receptors at the neuromuscular junction (NMJ). Also present at the NMJ are presynaptic nicotinic autoreceptors, and activation of these receptors enhances further ACh release. They are, unusually, positive rather than inhibitory, autoreceptors.

Clinical implications: Drugs which act at both muscarinic and nicotinic receptors are widely used clinically. Drugs which act to inhibit AChE, and so cause increased ACh levels, are also useful (see table, 'Drugs mimicking or effecting acetylcholine transmission').

Drugs mimicking or effecting acetylcholine transmission

Drug	Action	Clinical use
Atropine (injection)	Muscarinic antagonist	Treatment of bradycardias
Ipratropium bromide (inhaler)	Antimuscarinic which prevents secretion from bronchial epithelia	Asthma or chronic bronchitis
Neostigmine	Acetylcholine esterase inhibitor	Reversal of nondepolarised neuromuscular blockade
Suxamethonium	Agonist at nicotinic receptors causing depolarising block	Neuromuscular blocking agent (depolarising)
Dicyclomine (oral)	Antimuscarinic which causes reduced GI motility	Irritable bowel syndrome
Vecuronium (injection)	Nicotinic antagonist at the NMJ causing nondepolarising blockade	Nondepolarising neuromuscular blocking
Atropine (eye drops)	Dilate the pupil	Examination of the eye

FIG. 8.1 The synthesis and breakdown of ACh

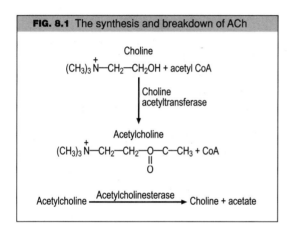

Choline

$$(CH_3)_3 \overset{+}{N}-CH_2-CH_2OH + acetyl\ CoA$$

Choline acetyltransferase

Acetylcholine

$$(CH_3)_3 \overset{+}{N}-CH_2-CH_2-O-\underset{\underset{O}{\|}}{C}-CH_3 + CoA$$

Acetylcholine $\xrightarrow{\text{Acetylcholinesterase}}$ Choline + acetate

REVISION AID
Acetylcholine

- Acetylcholine is synthesised in the nerve terminal, from choline by choline acetyltransferase. It is broken down and inactivated in the synaptic cleft by acetylcholinesterase

- Acetylcholine is often cotransmitted with peptide neurotransmitters

- Acetylcholine acts on two types of receptors: muscarinic and nicotinic

- Muscarinic M_1, M_3 and M_5 receptors act via Gq/11 to stimulate inositol 1,4,5-triphosphate (IP_3), whereas M_2 and M_4 receptors act via Gi/o to inhibit adenylyl cyclase

- Muscarinic receptors are G-protein-linked; nicotinic receptors are receptor-operated cation channels

- ACh is the neurotransmitter at the ganglia of the parasympathetic and sympathetic systems

- ACh is the postganglionic transmitter in the parasympathetic system

FIG. 8.2 The role of ACh in the peripheral nervous system

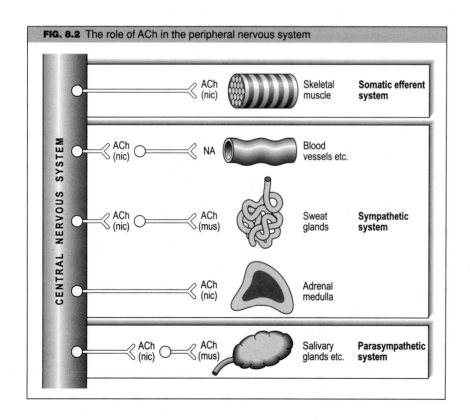

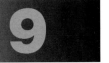

Noradrenaline

Biochemistry: Noradrenaline is synthesised from L-tyrosine. Tyrosine is taken up by the cell and then converted to DOPA (dihydroxyphenylalanine). This in turn is converted into dopamine by DOPA decarboxylase and finally into noradrenaline by dopamine-β-hydroxylase. Tyrosine hydroxylase regulates the rate-limiting step in this chain, and noradrenaline can inhibit tyrosine hydroxylase. Hence, noradrenaline can inhibit its own synthesis.

In the adrenal medulla, another enzyme is present, phenylethanolamine N-methyl transferase (PNMT), which converts noradrenaline into adrenaline.

Noradrenaline is stored in vesicles, along with ATP (also a transmitter) and a protein, chromogranin A. Dopamine-β-hydroxylase is also found in the vesicle. Neuropeptide Y (NPY), a peptide transmitter, may also be stored with noradrenaline.

Once released the noradrenaline is inactivated by reuptake back into the nerve terminal and surrounding cells. There are two uptake systems. Uptake system 1 is found on noradrenergic terminals and has a high specificity and affinity for noradrenaline. Surrounding cells (i.e. glial cells) have uptake system 2 with a lower specificity and affinity for noradrenaline but a higher capacity.

Once inside a cell, noradrenaline is metabolised by two enzymes: monoamine oxidase A (MAO_A) and catechol-O-methyl transferase (COMT). The eventual product of these enzymes can be either 3-methoxy-4-hydroxymandelic acid (VMA) formed mainly in the periphery, or 3-methoxy, 4-hydroxyphenylglycol (MOPEG), formed mainly in the CNS.

Noradrenaline receptors and distribution: Noradrenaline is an important transmitter in both the CNS and the autonomic nervous system. It is the major transmitter released by the postganglionic neurons of the sympathetic system, and has a wide range of effects.

Noradrenaline increases the rate and force of the action of the heart (through β_1 receptors). It generally causes constriction, however, in blood vessels (through α receptors), although it can cause dilation (through β_2 receptors).

In the CNS the most distinct group of noradrenergic neurons is the locus ceruleus which is found in the pons. These neurons project, via the dorsal noradrenergic bundle, to innervate large areas of the cortex, cerebellum and hippocampus. Other groups of noradrenergic neurons project via the ventral noradrenergic bundle to the hypothalamus, hippocampus, cerebellum and spinal cord.

Noradrenaline can act on both α and β adrenoreceptors although it is much more potent on α receptors. There are multiple types of each of these receptors: two groups of α receptors, α_1 (including subtypes 1A, 1B and 1C) and α_2 (including subtypes 2A, 2B and 2C), and three groups of β receptors β_1, β_2, and β_3. They are all G-protein-linked receptors; α_1 receptors couple to Gq/11 and stimulate IP_3/DAG production; α_2 receptors couple to Gi/o and decrease cAMP (they are often presynaptic autoregulatory receptors), whilst β receptors couple to Gs and increase cAMP synthesis. The β_3 receptor is found in brown adipose tissue, and stimulates the production of heat.

Clinical implications: Noradrenaline itself is rarely used clinically, although many therapeutic drugs that manipulate noradrenaline levels or act on adrenoceptors are used. Adrenaline is used in cardiac arrest and anaphylactic shock. The β_1 agonist, dobutamine, is used in cardiogenic shock, whilst the β_2 agonist, salbutamol, is commonly used in inhalers for the treatment of asthma. The α agonist, phenylephedrine, is used to treat hypotension after spinal or epidural anaesthesia. Drugs which block β adrenoceptors (e.g. propanolol) are used for a variety of ailments, e.g. the treatment of hypertension, arrhythmias, anxiety and to prevent myocardial infarction. Topical administration of timolol is used in glaucoma.

FIG. 9.1 Biosynthesis of catecholamines

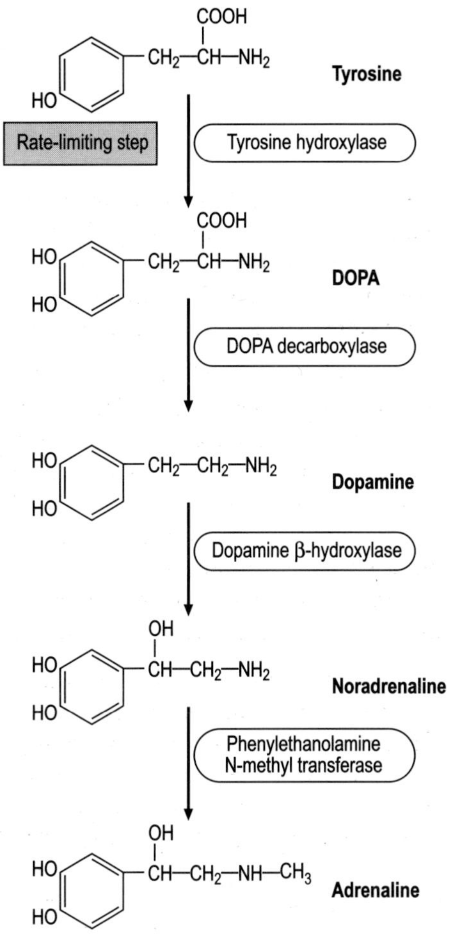

$$CH_2-CH-NH_2 \quad COOH$$

Tyrosine

Rate-limiting step → (Tyrosine hydroxylase)

$$CH_2-CH-NH_2 \quad COOH$$

DOPA

(DOPA decarboxylase)

$$CH_2-CH_2-NH_2$$

Dopamine

(Dopamine β-hydroxylase)

$$CH-CH_2-NH_2 \quad OH$$

Noradrenaline

(Phenylethanolamine N-methyl transferase)

$$CH-CH_2-NH-CH_3 \quad OH$$

Adrenaline

REVISION AID
Noradrenaline

- Noradrenaline is synthesised from L-tyrosine via a multistep process

- It is stored with other transmitters such as ATP and sometimes NPY

- Its action is terminated by reuptake

- It is broken down by MAO and COMT into VMA (periphery) or MOPEG (CNS)

- It is the main postganglionic transmitter for the sympathetic nervous system

- In the CNS the main body of noradrenergic neurons is the locus ceruleus; noradrenergic neurons diffusely innervate large areas of the brain, e.g. cortex, cerebellum, hypothalamus and hippocampus

- It is more potent at α receptors than β receptors

- There are multiple adrenoceptors: α_{1A-C}, α_{2A-C}, β_1, β_2 and β_3

FIG. 9.2 Main noradrenergic pathways in the CNS

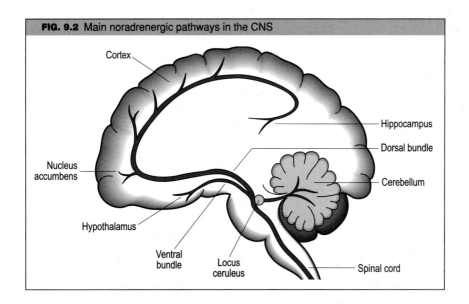

Cortex

Hippocampus

Dorsal bundle

Cerebellum

Nucleus accumbens

Hypothalamus

Ventral bundle

Locus ceruleus

Spinal cord

10 Dopamine

Biochemistry: Dopamine is synthesised from tyrosine via DOPA (dihydroxyphenylalanine) by tyrosine hydroxylase and DOPA decarboxylase. In many neurons dopamine is then converted into noradrenaline. However dopamine is an important neurotransmitter in its own right. Following neuronal release it is inactivated by a specific reuptake system. Dopamine is metabolised by monoamine oxidase (MAO) and catechol-O-methyl transferase (COMT). The major metabolites are 3,4-hydroxyphenylacetic acid (DOPAC) and homovanillic acid (HVA).

MPTP (1-methyl-4-phenyl-1,2,3,6-tetrahydropyridine) specifically kills dopaminergic neurons to produce animal models of parkinsonism. MPTP is selectively taken up by dopaminergic neurons and metabolised to the toxic product MPP$^+$ by MAO type B (MAO$_B$).

Dopamine receptors and distribution:
Five dopamine receptor genes have been sequenced. D_1 and D_5 couple via Gs to activate adenylyl cyclase, while D_2, D_3 and D_4 couple to Gi and inhibit adenylyl cylase.

There are three major dopaminergic pathways in the CNS:

1. The nigrostriatal pathway projects from the substantia nigra (midbrain) to the caudate nucleus and putamen (the striatum). It forms part of the extrapyramidal system and controls voluntary movements. Dopamine inhibits excitatory cholinergic and inhibitory GABA-ergic neurons in the striatum. Loss of dopaminergic neurons in the substantia nigra causes parkinsonism.

2. The mesolimbic (and mesocortical) pathway projects from the ventral tegmentum of the midbrain to many sites in the limbic system and cortex. These projections are associated with reward and mood, and may become overactive in psychoses such as schizophrenia. Many addictive drugs may modulate the function of this pathway (particularly its projections to the nucleus accumbens).

3. The tuberoinfundibular system projects from the arcuate nucleus of the hypothalamus to the median eminence in the hypothalamus. This pathway inhibits prolactin release and regulates lactation and fertility.

Peripheral dopamine receptors in the gut and renal vasculature produce selective vasodilation and increase renal blood flow.

Clinical implications: Drugs which facilitate dopaminergic transmission are used to treat parkinsonism. Examples include the dopamine precursor, levodopa (L-dopa), dopamine agonists and MAO type B inhibitors. They can cause hallucinations, depression, nausea, vomiting and other movement disorders.

Dopamine antagonists, such as chlorpromazine, are used to treat psychoses such as schizophrenia. Side-effects include movement disorders, drowsiness, infertility and galactorrhoea (excessive lactation). Dopamine agonists are also used as antiemetics, to suppress lactation and treat infertility (due to hyperprolactinaemia). Dopamine infusions are used to produce renal vasodilation and prevent renal failure in shock (low blood pressure in severely ill patients).

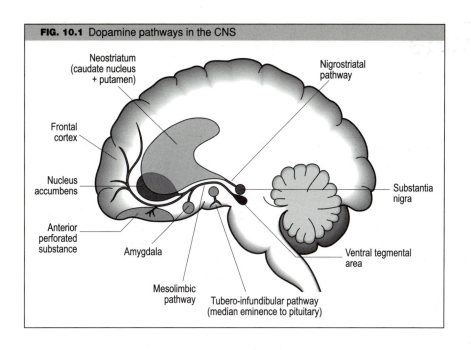

FIG. 10.1 Dopamine pathways in the CNS

Neostriatum
(caudate nucleus
+ putamen)

Nigrostriatal
pathway

Frontal
cortex

Nucleus
accumbens

Substantia
nigra

Anterior
perforated
substance

Amygdala

Ventral tegmental
area

Mesolimbic
pathway

Tubero-infundibular pathway
(median eminence to pituitary)

Drugs which affect dopaminergic transmission	
Drug	**Comment**
Levodopa (DOPA)	Dopamine precursor used in parkinsonism
Bromocriptine	Dopamine antagonist used in parkinsonism, also to suppress lactation, and to treat infertility due to hyperprolactinaemia
Selegiline	MAO_B inhibitor used in parkinsonism
Domperidone	Dopamine antagonist used as antiemetic
Antipsychotics e.g. **chlorpromazine**	Dopamine antagonists
Amphetamine	Displaces dopamine from storage vesicles, prevents metabolism and reuptake. Used illicitly, and for obesity, and in hyperactive children
Tricylic antidepressants and **cocaine**	Prevent dopamine and noradrenaline reuptake
Monoamine oxidase inhibitors	Prevent dopamine and noradrenaline metabolism. Used in depression. Toxic interaction with food and other drugs
Tetrabenazine	Disrupts dopamine storage. Used in Huntington's chorea

REVISION AID

Dopamine

- Dopamine is synthesised from tyrosine via DOPA. It may be converted to noradrenaline but is also an important neurotransmitter in its own right

- There are five genes for dopamine receptors: D_1 and D_5 activate cAMP synthesis, and D_2, D_3 and D_4 inhibit cAMP synthesis

- There are three dopaminergic pathways in the central nervous system: the nigrostriatal pathway (which becomes inactive in parkinsonism); the mesolimbic pathway (which becomes overactive in schizophrenia), and the tuberoinfundibular pathway (which regulates prolactin release)

- Drugs which facilitate dopaminergic transmission are used to treat parkinsonism. They can cause hallucinations, depression, nausea and vomiting

- Dopamine antagonists are used to treat schizophrenia and other psychoses. They produce movement disorders and drowsiness

- Amphetamine, cocaine and other addictive drugs facilitate dopaminergic and noradrenergic transmission

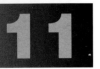

5-Hydroxytryptamine

Biochemistry: 5-Hydroxytryptamine (5-HT, also called serotonin) is synthesised from L-tryptophan via 5-hydroxytryptophan by tryptophan hydroxylase and dopa decarboxylase (L-aromatic acid decarboxylase). It is an important neurotransmitter in the CNS and is often stored with various peptide hormones such as substance P. 5-HT is also found in high concentrations in the wall of the intestine and in platelets.

The action of 5-HT is terminated by reuptake (by a high affinity 5-HT-specific system). In the presynaptic terminal, free 5-HT (which has not been recycled into vesicles) is metabolised by monoamine oxidase (MAO) and aldehyde dehydrogenase. The main metabolite is 5-hydroxyindoleacetic acid (5-HIAA).

5-HT receptors and distribution: At present seven families of 5-HT receptors have been identified: 5-HT_{1-7}. 5-HT_3 receptors are unusual as they couple to a cation channel, whilst the other families of 5-HT receptors all couple to G-proteins.

There are two main pathways of 5-HT-containing neurons in the CNS. One pathway, originating from the raphe nucleus, innervates various parts of the brain (see Fig. 11.1). The second pathway originates in the brain stem and extends axons to the spinal cord.

5-HT has an important role in the periphery. In blood vessels 5-HT can act both as a vasodilator (on arterioles) and as a vasoconstrictor (on large arteries). The effects of 5-HT are therefore dependent on the type of receptor present in a blood vessel. The 5-HT_1 and 5-HT_2 receptors are thought to be responsible for vasodilation and vasoconstriction, respectively. Also, 5-HT is involved in gastrointestinal peristalsis, can stimulate platelet aggregation and can act to stimulate pain fibres.

Clinical implications: Drugs that affect 5-HT systems are used to treat a wide range of conditions including, depression, anxiety, migraine, obsessive-compulsive disorders and cytotoxic-induced nausea.

Blockers of 5-HT reuptake are used in the treatment of depression. These include the SSRIs (serotonin selective reuptake inhibitors) such as fluoxetine (Prozac).

Buspirone, a 5-HT_{1A} partial agonist, is used as an anxiolytic, and sumatriptan, a 5-HT_{1D} agonist, is used in the treatment of migraines. Ondansetron a specific 5-HT_3 antagonist, is a powerful (and expensive) antiemetic. The hallucinogenic drug, LSD, is a 5-HT_2 partial agonist.

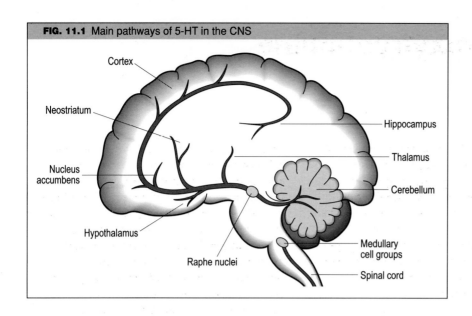

FIG. 11.1 Main pathways of 5-HT in the CNS

Cortex

Neostriatum

Nucleus accumbens

Hypothalamus

Raphe nuclei

Hippocampus

Thalamus

Cerebellum

Medullary cell groups

Spinal cord

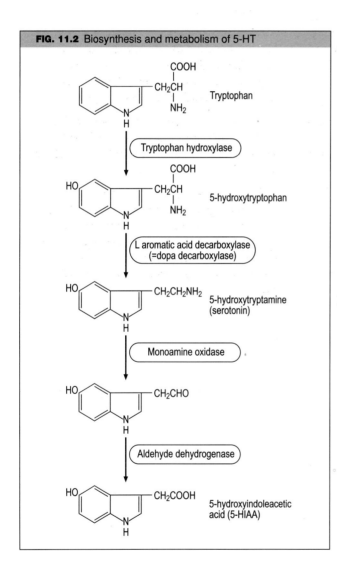

FIG. 11.2 Biosynthesis and metabolism of 5-HT

Tryptophan

Tryptophan hydroxylase

5-hydroxytryptophan

L aromatic acid decarboxylase (=dopa decarboxylase)

5-hydroxytryptamine (serotonin)

Monoamine oxidase

Aldehyde dehydrogenase

5-hydroxyindoleacetic acid (5-HIAA)

5-HT receptors

5-HT receptor type	Effector	Effect
1A, 1B, 1D, 1E, 1F	Gi/o	$\downarrow$ cAMP
2A, 2B, 2C	Gq/11	$\uparrow$ IP$_3$/DAG
3	Cation channel	$\uparrow$ Na$^+$ > Ca^{2+} > K$^+$
4	Gs	$\uparrow$ cAMP
5A, 5B	Unknown	Unknown
6	Gs	$\uparrow$ cAMP
7	Gs	$\uparrow$ cAMP

REVISION AID
5-HT

- 5-HT (serotonin) is synthesised from tryptophan via 5-hydroxytryptophan

- At present seven groups of 5-HT receptors are known, all of which are G-protein-coupled, except for the 5-HT$_3$ receptor, which is a cation channel

- 5-HT is a neurotransmitter in the brain, spinal cord and myenteric plexus. It is also released as a local hormone in some parts of the periphery

- Drugs which block 5-HT reuptake are used in the treatment of depression

- Specific agonists and antagonists are used in the treatment of migraine and vomiting

12 GABA

Biochemistry: GABA (gamma-aminobutyric acid) is formed from glutamate by the enzyme glutamic acid decarboxylase. Once it is released, specific reuptake systems remove the GABA into surrounding cells, where it can be broken down by GABA transaminase into succinic semialdehyde, which in its turn can be broken down to succinic acid or restored for further release. GABA is the major inhibitory transmitter in the CNS. The vast majority of central neurons possess GABA receptors. GABA is most commonly found in short interneurons, although there are some longer neurons running to the cerebellum and the striatum.

GABA-ergic receptors and distribution:
There are two families of GABA receptors: $GABA_A$ receptors are linked to ion channels, whilst $GABA_B$ receptors are G-protein receptors linked to Gi/o.

The $GABA_A$ receptor consists of five subunits. Activation of this channel causes an influx of Cl^- ions. Six α, four β, four γ, one δ and two ρ subunits have been so far described. Channels are made up of different combinations of these subunits and show distinct distribution and pharmacological properties. For instance, alcohol can enhance the action of GABA providing the $\gamma 2L$ subunit is present.

$GABA_A$ receptors are in general selectively activated by muscimol and inhibited by the competitive antagonist bicuculline. In addition to the GABA site, there are also modulatory sites. Benzodiazepines bind to one of these modulatory sites, and enhance GABA's action by increasing the affinity of the receptor for GABA and by increasing the probability that the channel will open. Barbiturates can also bind to $GABA_A$ receptors at a different site from benzodiazepines. They also can enhance GABA's action by increasing its affinity for the receptor and also by increasing the duration of time for which a channel is open. Other modulatory sites exist for alcohol, some anaesthetics and steroid hormones.

Flumazenil is a competitive antagonist at the benzodiazepine site, and indeed benzodiazepines and barbiturates exist which inhibit GABA's action. These agents are termed *inverse* agonists.

$GABA_B$ receptors are G-protein-linked receptors and can be activated by baclofen and inhibited by the selective antagonist, phaclofen. They are found presynaptically whereas $GABA_A$ receptors are mainly postsynaptic. Activation of $GABA_B$ receptors causes a decreased Ca^{2+} and an increased K^+ conductance in the cell.

Clinical implications: Benzodiazepines, such as temazepam, are commonly used to treat insomnia, anxiety, alcohol withdrawal, spasticity and as premedication (administered before an operation). Benzodiazepines and barbiturates (rarely) are sometimes used as antiepileptics. Vigabatrin, which inhibits GABA transaminase and so elevates GABA levels, is an antiepileptic. The $GABA_B$ agonist, baclofen, is also used as a muscle relaxant in spasticity.

FIG. 12.1 A simplified model of GABA release and uptake, and the GABA$_A$ receptor

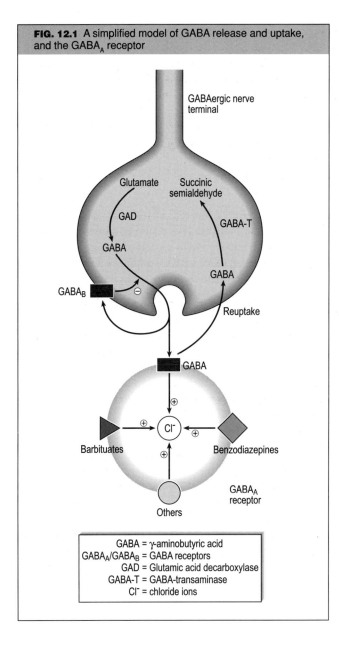

GABAergic nerve terminal

Glutamate

Succinic semialdehyde

GAD

GABA-T

GABA

GABA

GABA$_B$

⊖

Reuptake

GABA

⊕

Cl⁻

⊕ ⊕

Barbituates

Benzodiazepines

⊕

GABA$_A$ receptor

Others

GABA = γ-aminobutyric acid
GABA$_A$/GABA$_B$ = GABA receptors
GAD = Glutamic acid decarboxylase
GABA-T = GABA-transaminase
Cl⁻ = chloride ions

GABA (gamma-aminobutyric acid)

- GABA is synthesised by glutamic acid decarboxylase and broken down by GABA transaminase

- GABA is a neurotransmitter in one-third of all synapses in the CNS

- GABA is the principal inhibitory neurotransmitter in the CNS; most neurons have GABA receptors

- GABA is not found in the periphery, although GABA receptors are sometimes present

- GABA$_A$ receptors contain Cl⁻ channels and have modulatory sites for benzodiazepines, barbiturates, alcohol, anaesthetics and steroids

- GABA$_B$ receptors are presynaptic and are G-protein-linked

- Benzodiazepines and barbiturates enhance the action of GABA

13 Histamine and prostanoids

Histamine

Histamine is synthesised by histidine decarboxylase from histidine. It is broken down by histaminase and by N-methyl-transferase (which adds a methyl group). At present there are three known types of histamine receptor: H_1, H_2 and H_3. The first two receptors are G-protein-linked; H_1 receptors are Gq/11-linked and stimulate the production of IP_3/DAG, and H_2 receptors are Gs-linked and stimulate the production of cAMP. The nature of the H_3 receptor is still unknown.

Histamine has an important role in inflammatory processes. It is stored in mast cells and basophils and is released during anaphylactic shock. It causes the *triple response* when injected into the skin; this comprises local vasodilation of small arterioles, weals because of increased permeability of postcapillary venules and reddening, or flare, through antidromic stimulation of sensory fibres. There is little histidine decarboxylase in mast cells and basophils, so histamine stores refill slowly. Some drugs such as morphine can cause release of histamine and so can cause allergic reactions. Histamine acts via H_1 receptors to contract bronchial and other smooth muscle and dilate blood vessels. It also increases cardiac rate and output via cardiac H_2 receptors. The actions at the H_1 receptors can be blocked by antagonists such as mepyramine (termed 'antihistamines'). Histamine acts in the stomach via H_2 receptors to cause release of gastric acid. These receptors are a prime target in the treatment of peptic ulcers where H_2 antagonists can be used.

In addition to these peripheral effects histamine is also a neurotransmitter in the CNS. Histaminergic neurons originate from a small region in the hypothalamus and innervate large regions of the cortex and midbrain. The H_3 receptor is also found in the CNS where it is believed to have a presynaptic inhibitory effect.

Prostanoids

The term 'prostanoids' encompasses prostaglandins and thromboxanes. These compounds are not stored in vesicles but are synthesised when required. The precursor for prostanoids is arachidonic acid (an unsaturated fatty acid) which is released by hydrolysis of phospholipids by phospholipase A_2. Two forms of phospholipase A_2 exist, one in the intracellular cytosol, which is believed to mediate the inflammatory role of prostanoids, the other in the extracellular fluid. Phospholipase D and phospholipase C can also help to produce arachidonate acid (via a two-step pathway). Arachidonate acid is then further metabolised by cyclooxygenase (COX) into prostaglandins and thromboxanes. PGI_2 (prostacyclin), PGE_2, PGD_2, $PGF_{2\alpha}$ and TXA_2 are the main prostanoids.

Cyclooxygenase has two distinct types: COX_1 is found in most cells and is always present, whilst COX_2 is induced in inflammatory cells by various stimuli. COX produces the prostaglandin PGH_2, which is then further metabolised into different prostanoids depending on the cell type, e.g. mast cells synthesise PGD_2 whilst vascular endothelium synthesises mainly prostacyclin. Prostanoid actions are terminated by reuptake and rapid metabolism by prostaglandin-specific enzymes and also by nonspecific fatty acid metabolising enzymes. High concentrations of these prostaglandin-specific enzymes exist in the lung. Prostacyclin and TXA_2 are not taken up by cells but are rapidly broken down in the plasma (the $t_{\frac{1}{2}}$ is less than a minute for these compounds compared with approximately 5 minutes for other prostanoids).

At present five distinct classes of prostanoid receptors are known. Many further subtypes also exist; all those described to date are G-protein-linked. The actions of prostanoids are varied and depend on the exact prostanoid and receptor present. (See the table 'Prostanoids'.)

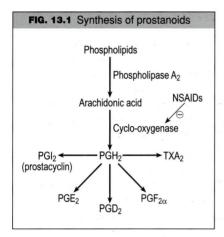

FIG. 13.1 Synthesis of prostanoids

Prostanoids

Prostanoid	Receptor	Intracellular mechanism	Action
PGD_2	DP	↑ cAMP	Vasodilation; inhibition of platelet aggregation
$PGF_{2\alpha}$	FP	↑ DAG/IP_3	Myometrial contraction
PGI_2 (prostacyclin)	IP	↑ cAMP	Vasodilation; inhibition of platelet aggregation
TXA_2	TP	↑ DAG/IP_3	Vasoconstriction; platelet aggregation
PGE_2	EP_1	↑ DAG/IP_3	Contraction of bronchial and gastrointestinal smooth muscle
	EP_2	↑ cAMP	Broncho- and vasodilation
	EP_3	↓ cAMP or ↑ DAG/IP_3	Contraction of intestinal muscle; inhibition of gastric acid secretion; stimulation of gastric mucus secretion

14 Excitatory amino acids and opioid peptides

Excitatory amino acids (EAAs)

Glutamate, an amino acid which is formed as part of the Krebs cycle, is also a transmitter and has its own receptors. Glutamate is stored in its own synaptic vesicles which are distinct from any other stores. It is released by neurons and its action is terminated by reuptake into glial cells. It is then converted to glutamine and recirculated to neurons. There are three broad classes of glutamate receptors: metabotropic receptors, NMDA (N-methyl-D-aspartate) receptors and AMPA (α-amino-3-hydroxy-5-methyl-isoxazole)/ kainate receptors.

The metabotropic glutamate receptors (mGluRs), are linked to G-proteins and are subdivided into three groups. Group 1 includes mGluRs 1 and 5, group 2 includes mGluRs 2 and 3, whilst group 3 includes mGluRs 4, 6, 7 and 8.

The AMPA/kainate and the NMDA receptors are all receptor-operated cation channels which allow the influx of Na^+ and Ca^{2+}. The AMPA/kainate receptors are made up of different subunit combinations. The subunits specify the receptor selectivity; some receptors are AMPA-preferring (made up of subunits Glu 1, 2, 3 and 4), others are kainate-preferring (made up of subunits Glu 5, 6 and 7, or Ka 1 and 2).

The NMDA receptors are also made up of five different subunit combinations (subunits nmda 1 and nmda 2A–2D). Glycine is termed a co-agonist at the NMDA receptor, as glycine must bind to a distinct modulatory site on the NMDA receptor for the ion channel to open in response to glutamate.

At present there are no drugs which act at EAA receptors, although such drugs are being developed. Antagonists at these receptors may prove useful in the treatment of strokes. Strokes cause neurons to die and release large amounts of glutamate. The surrounding neurons are stimulated by this glutamate, causing a large increase in Ca^{2+} which can lead to further cell death. A glutamate antagonist could prevent this.

Aspartate is another amino acid which can also be formed from the Krebs cycle. It may also have a neurotransmitter role, and can stimulate some glutamate receptors.

Opioid peptides

Opioids are drugs which produce morphine-like effects, whose action can be reversed by the opioid antagonist, naloxone. Opiates are naturally occurring morphine-like drugs found in the opium poppy (*Papaver somniferum*). Endogenous opioids are peptides, and are synthesised from large precursor peptides, which are cleaved into smaller active fragments. There are four main endogenous opioid peptides: β-endorphin, dynorphin, leucine-enkephalin (leu-enkephalin) and methionine-enkephalin (met-enkephalin). These peptides may have additional amino acids tagged onto the end of their C-terminus. There are three pecursor peptides.

1. Proenkephalin contains met- and leu-enkephalin and several extended forms of met-enkephalin.
2. Prodynorphin contains dynorphin, leu-enkephalin and several extended forms of leu-enkephalin.
3. Proopiomelanocortin contains β-endorphin and also melanocyte-stimulating hormone (MSH) and ACTH (corticotrophin).

There are three opioid receptors (μ, δ, κ) all of which are linked to the G-protein Gi/o. They are found in the CNS and the gastrointestinal tract. All opioid receptors are stimulated endogenously by β-endorphin. The enkephalins preferentially stimulate the δ receptors and dynorphin preferentially stimulates the κ receptor. Morphine is an agonist with a potency order of $\mu > \kappa > \delta$ opioid receptors.

Opioids are used as analgesics, antidiarrhoeals and antitussives. Methadone is used in withdrawal treatment of opioid addicts. The antagonist naloxone is used to reverse opioid overdoses.

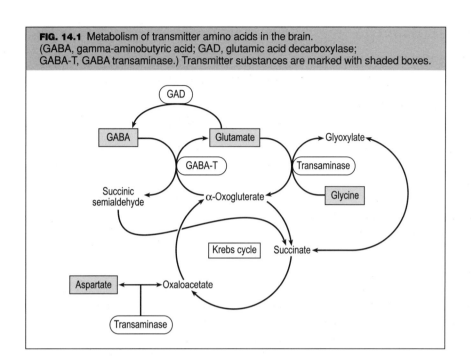

FIG. 14.1 Metabolism of transmitter amino acids in the brain. (GABA, gamma-aminobutyric acid; GAD, glutamic acid decarboxylase; GABA-T, GABA transaminase.) Transmitter substances are marked with shaded boxes.

Opioid effects

Therapeutic effects	Unwanted effects
Analgesia	Euphoria
Euphoria	Respiratory depression
Constipation	Narcosis
Antitussive	Tolerance
	Physical dependence
	Nausea
	Constipation

Excitatory amino acids (EAAs)

- Glutamate is an excitatory neurotransmitter

- There are three main types of EAA receptor: metabotropic, NMDA and AMPA/kainate

- Aspartate, another amino acid, can activate the NMDA and AMPA receptor

- These amino acids are often referred to as excitatory amino acids (EAAs)

Opioids

- Opioids are drugs which have similar actions to morphine and whose effects can be reversed by the opioid antagonist, naloxone

- There are four main opioid peptides: leu-enkephalin, met-enkephalin, dynorphin and β-endorphin

- They are synthesised as large peptide precursors which are then cleaved to release the opioid peptides and other peptide hormones such as ACTH and MSH

- There are three precursor peptides: proenkephalin, prodynorphin and proopiomelanocortin

- Opioid receptors are all G-protein-linked. They increase K^+ conductance and reduce Ca^{2+} conductance and cAMP levels

- Morphine and codeine are commonly used opioids

15 Purinergic transmission and neurotransmitter transporters

Purinergic transmission

ATP (the prototypical energy source of the body) is also a neurotransmitter. ATP is stored as a cotransmitter in both noradrenergic and cholinergic neurons and when it is released, acts at specific receptors termed the P_2 purinoceptors. Its action is often much quicker than that of noradrenaline or acetylcholine. In addition the metabolites of ATP (ADP and AMP) can act at these receptors.

Five classes of P_2 receptors have been identified so far. The P_{2T}, P_{2X} and P_{2Z} receptors are linked to a cation channel, whilst P_{2U} and P_{2Y} are G-protein-linked receptors which activate Gq/11.

The second class of purinoceptors is the P_1 receptors. They are activated by adenosine, which can be released by cells or produced by the breakdown of ATP. Rather than being used as a neurotransmitter, adenosine is thought to act as a local hormone. Adenosine receptors are found on many peripheral tissues as well as in the CNS. Adenosine's action is terminated by further breakdown or by reuptake via a specific system. At present, four classes of adenosine receptors are known: A_1, A_{2A}, A_{2B} and A_3. They are all linked to G-proteins.

The actions of both ATP and adenosine are wide and varied, and drugs acting on these receptors are presently being developed. However, the only clinically used drug is adenosine itself which is sometimes administered for dysrhythmias.

Neurotransmitter reuptake systems

Specific neurotransmitter transporters have been identified for dopamine, noradrenaline, 5-HT, glutamate, aspartate, GABA, glycine, adenosine, and many other important molecules, including choline. These transporters are located within the synaptic membranes of neurons that use the particular transmitter. They are probably the most important mechanism for terminating synaptic transmission (except in the case of acetylcholine which is inactivated in the synaptic cleft by acetylcholinesterase). Neurotransmitter uptake systems are cotransporters (symporters) which also transport sodium (and often chloride) ions with the neurotransmitter. Hence the energy stored in the transmembrane electrochemical gradients drives the reuptake of the neurotransmitters. Tricyclic antidepressants and stimulant drugs (such as cocaine and amphetamine) inhibit these neurotransmitter transporters.

The uptake system for catecholamines has been well studied. There are two systems, uptake 1 and uptake 2. Uptake 1 has a high specificity for noradrenaline and is found on noradrenergic neurons; uptake 2 is found on other cell types and has a lower specificity but a higher capacity. (See the table 'Catecholamine transporters'.)

Catecholamine transporters

	Uptake 1	Uptake 2
Characteristics	High specificity	Low specificity
	Low capacity	High capacity
Location	Neuronal	Nonneuronal
Substrates	Noradrenaline	Noradrenaline
	Dopamine	Dopamine
	5-HT	5-HT
		Histamine
Inhibitor	Cocaine	Some steroid hormones
	Amphetamine	
	Tricyclic depressants	

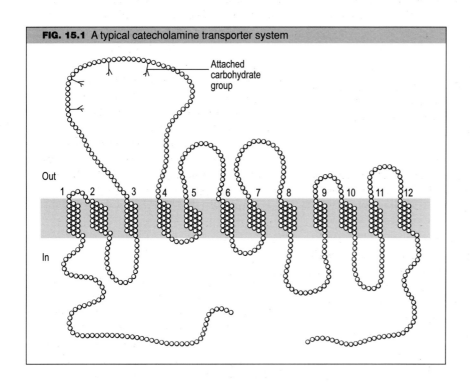

FIG. 15.1 A typical catecholamine transporter system

Purinergic receptors

Receptor	Effector	Effect
P_{2T}, P_{2X}, P_{2Z}	Cation channel	$\uparrow Na^+ > Ca^{2+} > K^+$
P_{2U}, P_{2Y}	Gq/11	$\uparrow IP_3$/DAG
A_1, A_3	Gi/o	$\downarrow$ cAMP
A_{2A}, A_{2B}	Gs	$\uparrow$ cAMP

16 Diuretics: frusemide and bendrofluazide

Diuretics act on the kidney to produce an initial increase in urine output. Several also have vasodilator actions at subdiuretic doses. They are used widely to treat hypertension and heart failure. Only 5% of sodium reabsorption occurs in the distal convoluted tubule of the nephron. Consequently thiazides and potassium-sparing diuretics, which act on the distal tubule, produce only a mild diuresis.

Thiazide diuretics: bendrofluazide

Mechanism of action: Thiazide diuretics inhibit reabsorption of sodium (and chloride) in the distal nephron. Their cellular actions are uncertain. However, they directly inhibit a sodium–chloride cotransporter in the distal nephron. Thiazides also produce vasodilation by an uncertain extrarenal mechanism. This may account for their antihypertensive action.

Side-effects: Thiazide diuretics promote secretion of potassium ions. Prolonged treatment produces hypokalaemia which can be treated with potassium supplements or potassium-sparing diuretics. Thiazides may exacerbate diabetes mellitus and gout.

Potassium-sparing diuretics: spironolactone and amiloride

Mechanism of action: Spironolactone is an antagonist of the hormone aldosterone. Aldosterone acts on intracellular receptors in cells of the distal tubule and collecting ducts, causing synthesis of membrane proteins which excrete potassium and reabsorb sodium ions. Spironolactone abolishes this effect, leading to potassium retention and sodium excretion.

Amiloride blocks sodium–hydrogen exchange transporters and sodium channels in the distal nephron. These systems allow sodium entry into the cells from the tubule and reabsorption. Hence amiloride prevents sodium reabsorption. Sodium ions in cells of the distal tubule are also exchanged for potassium ions in the blood. The potassium is then secreted. Amiloride prevents this exchange, leading to retention of potassium.

Side-effects: Potassium-sparing diuretics are usually combined with other diuretics (which cause potassium excretion). However, they can produce hyperkalaemia when used alone.

Loop diuretics: frusemide

Mechanism of action: These are the most potent diuretics. They prevent the reabsorption of sodium and chloride from the ascending limb of the loop of Henle. This prevents water reabsorption from the collecting duct by osmosis. Loop diuretics also produce vasodilation, by an unknown mechanism, which explains their rapid action in acute heart failure. Their diuretic effect is partly due to renal artery vasodilation which increases the glomerular filtration rate.

Pharmacokinetics: Frusemide is given by slow intravenous injection for acute heart failure (bolus injection can cause hypotension and fainting). In hypertension and heart failure loop diuretics are taken orally first thing in the morning as they produce a sudden diuresis.

Side-effects: Potassium loss leading to hypokalaemia is common. Consequently loop diuretics are often given with potassium-sparing agents or potassium supplements. They may cause hypovolaemia and hypotension, especially in elderly or dehydrated patients.

Other side-effects of diuretics

Less common side-effects of diuretics from any group include: acid–base imbalance, depletion states of ions such as calcium, magnesium and sodium. Gastrointestinal disturbances, pancreatitis, blood dyscrasia, allergic reactions, hearing loss (ototoxicity) and renal damage may also develop.

Mechanism of action of diuretics

Agent	Diuretic action	Antihypertensive action
Thiazides	Blocks Na$^+$/Cl$^-$ cotransporter in distal nephron	? Alter sodium and chloride utilisation in smooth muscle
Spironolactone (aldosterone antagonist)	Prevents synthesis of Na$^+$/K$^+$–ATPase antiport and Na$^+$ and K$^+$ channels in distal nephron	Not useful
Amiloride	Blocks Na$^+$/H$^+$ exchange and luminal sodium channels in distal nephron	Not useful
Loop diuretics	Block Na$^+$/2Cl$^-$/K$^+$ cotransporter in ascending loop of Henle	? Promotes renal prostaglandin release ? Alters smooth muscle sodium or calcium utilisation

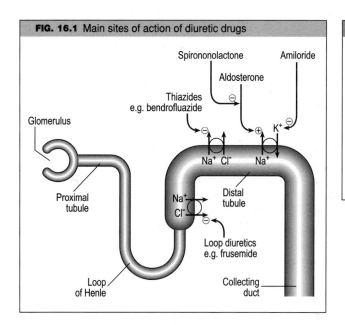

FIG. 16.1 Main sites of action of diuretic drugs

Osmotic diuretics

These agents are not used in cardiovascular disease. Mannitol is the only osmotic diuretic in use today. It is a simple carbohydrate which cannot cross cell membranes and has few cellular actions. However, it is filtered by the glomerulus but cannot be reabsorbed by the renal tubules. Hence, mannitol increases the solute concentration of the glomerular filtrate and produces an increase in urine volume by its osmotic effect. Mannitol is used to prevent or treat cerebral oedema after head injuries and during neurosurgical operations. Mannitol is also used to reduce corneal oedema in episodes of acute glaucoma (see Ch. 44).

REVISION AID
Diuretics

- Diuretics act on the kidney to produce an initial increase in urine output

- Diuretics are widely used to treat heart failure

- Thiazide diuretics, such as bendrofluazide, inhibit reabsorption of sodium in the distal nephron

- Potassium-sparing diuretics include spironolactone (an aldosterone antagonist) and amiloride. They act on the distal tubule and collecting ducts to prevent sodium reabsorption and potassium excretion

- Loop diuretics, such as frusemide, prevent the reabsorption of sodium and chloride from the ascending limb of the loop of Henle

- Loop diuretics are used intravenously in acute heart failure

- Thiazides and loop diuretics are used in hypertension, often at subdiuretic doses. They produce vasodilation by an uncertain mechanism

- Thiazides and loop diuretics can produce hypokalaemia and are often combined with potassium-sparing diuretics or potassium supplements

17 Beta-blockers: propranolol and atenolol

Beta-blockers (β-blockers) are antagonists of β-adrenergic receptors. They are used to treat hypertension, angina and cardiac arrhythmias. The β_1 receptors increase heart rate and cardiac muscle contractility, and β_2 receptors produce bronchodilation, vasodilation and glucose release from the liver. The catecholamines, noradrenaline and adrenaline, are agonists at these receptors. They are released from the sympathetic postganglionic nerve terminals and the adrenal medulla, during stress and exercise.

Mechanisms of action: The antihypertensive effect of β-blockers is poorly understood. Explanations include the following.

1. β-Blockers reduce heart rate and cardiac output possibly by blocking the effects of circulating catecholamines. There is an initial compensatory increase in peripheral resistance (due to the baroreceptor reflex) but this response gradually wanes. Hence cardiac output remains depressed while total peripheral resistance and blood pressure falls. The baroreceptor reflex becomes reset, probably by a central mechanism.

2. β-Blockers can reduce renin release from the kidneys. (Renin leads to synthesis of angiotensin II, a potent vasoconstrictor.) However, in many hypertensive patients changes in renin levels do not correlate well with the antihypertensive effects of β-blockers.

β-Blockers are useful intravenously in acute arrhythmias. They slow atrioventricular conduction and block the other arrhythmogenic effects of catecholamines. Some also block sodium channels in a similar manner to local anaesthetics.

β-Blockers are used in the prophylaxis of angina and after myocardial infarction to reduce infarct size and minimise the severity of subsequent infarcts. They reduce the unwanted effects of stress-induced catecholamine release such as increased heart rate and contractility, arrhythmogenesis and coronary vasoconstriction.

See the table 'Uses of beta-blockers' for other applications.

Side-effects: Many bronchodilators are β_2 agonists which are used to treat respiratory diseases. The older, unselective β-blockers, such as propranolol, prevent the therapeutic action of β_2 agonists and so impair treatment of bronchospasm. This is less of a problem with β_1-selective (or 'cardioselective') β-blockers, such as atenolol. However, even these agents have some β_2 antagonist properties. Hence all β-blockers are avoided in patients with respiratory diseases (e.g. asthma and chronic bronchitis).

β-Blockers reduce heart rate and contractility. This may worsen heart failure, produce fatigue and reduce exercise tolerance, and they may also cause bradycardias. β-Blockers produce uncomfortable cold hands and arms, especially in women, by occluding β-receptor-mediated vasodilation. However, β_1-selective agents may avoid this. Some β-blockers have intrinsic sympathomimetic activity (the capacity to stimulate as well as block adrenergic receptors). Use of these agents may avoid bradycardias and coldness of the extremities. β-Blockers are avoided in diabetics because they mask the warning signs of hypoglycaemia (sweating, palpitations and tremor).

Insomnia and depression occur with lipid-soluble β-blockers e.g. propranolol. Use of less lipid-soluble agents, e.g. atenolol, may avoid this.

Rebound angina can occur if β-blockers are stopped suddenly.

Uses of beta-blockers

Disorder	Mechanism of action
Hypertension (including preeclampsia and pregnancy-induced hypertension)	Reduced cardiac output Resetting of baroreceptor reflex Inhibition of renin release
Cardiac arrhythmias	Block arrhythmogenic effects of catecholamines
Myocardial infarction	Prevent catecholamine-induced coronary vasoconstriction and arrhythmias
Angina	Reduced cardiac output Prevent catecholamine-induced coronary vasoconstriction
Glaucoma	Reduce aqueous humour formation
Migraine prophylaxis	? Prevent cerebral vasodilation
Anxiety	Block peripheral signs of anxiety

Some drugs with multiple indications in cardiovascular disease

Drug	Biochemical actions	Selected physiological actions	Uses
Diuretics, e.g. bendrofluazide, frusemide	Various	Promote sodium excretion Venodilation Reduce TPR	Hypertension Heart failure Pulmonary oedema
β-Blockers, e.g. propranolol, atenolol	Catecholamine antagonist	Reduce renin secretion, heart rate, contractility and TPR Delay AV node conduction	Hypertension Arrhythmias Angina MI
Calcium channel blocker, e.g. nifedipine	Prevents L-type calcium channel opening	Delays AV node conduction Vasodilator	Hypertension Arrhythmias (SVT) Angina
ACE inhibitors, e.g. enalapril	Inhibit angiotensin II synthesis	Vasodilator Promote sodium secretion	Hypertension Heart failure
Nitrates, e.g. glyceryl trinitrate	Converted to nitric oxide	Vasodilator	Angina Heart failure
Digoxin	Promotes parasympathetic discharge to heart Inhibits Na^+/K^+ ATPase	Delays atrioventricular conduction Mild positive inotrope	Arrhythmias (SVT) Heart failure

TPR, total peripheral resistance; SVT, supraventricular tachycardia; MI, myocardial infarction; ACE, angiotensin-converting enzyme

REVISION AID
Beta-blockers

- β-Blockers, such as propranolol, are antagonists of β-adrenergic receptors

- Their antihypertensive effects involve reduction in cardiac output with resetting of the baroreceptor reflex and inhibition in renin release

- Other useful properties include the reduction of the unwanted effects of stress-induced catecholamine release, e.g. increased heart rate and contractility, arrhythmogenesis and coronary vasoconstriction

- They are useful in angina, acute cardiac arrhythmias and in the treatment and prevention of myocardial infarction

- β-Blockers must not be used in patients with asthma or other respiratory disorders, because they may cause bronchospasm and prevent the action of many bronchodilator drugs

- β-Blockers are avoided in severe heart failure because they reduce cardiac output

- β-Blockers are avoided in diabetics because they occlude the warning signs of hypoglycaemia

- Some side-effects may be avoided by using $β_1$-selective agents such as atenolol

18 Antihypertensive agents: nifedipine and enalapril

Hypertension (blood pressure consistently greater than 160/95 mmHg) causes cardiovascular disease, strokes and renal failure. Up to 20% of people over 45 years require antihypertensive drugs. There is no identifiable cause in 90% of patients. This *idiopathic hypertension* has a hereditary component. Somehow the baroreceptor reflex is reset to maintain blood pressure at a higher level and produce an increase in peripheral resistance. All antihypertensive drugs ultimately reduce peripheral resistance (although β-blockers also produce an initial fall in cardiac output).

Nondrug treatment of hypertension includes stopping smoking, taking regular exercise and reducing excessive weight and salt and alcohol intake. In 50% of patients drugs are also required. The four most widely used types of antihypertensives are diuretics, β-blockers, calcium channel blockers and angiotensin-converting enzyme (ACE) inhibitors.

Diuretics and β-blockers: Thiazide diuretics, such as bendrofluazide, are used at low doses in hypertension. Their mechanism of action in hypertension is uncertain. They cause hypokalaemia and may exacerbate diabetes and gout (see Ch. 50). Salt restriction is essential for their antihypertensive effects.

Similarly, with β-blockers, such as atenolol, the mechanism of action in hypertension is uncertain. Contraindications include respiratory disease, diabetes and heart failure (see Ch. 19). Diuretics and β-blockers have more side-effects than calcium channel blockers and ACE inhibitors, but are cheaper.

Calcium channel blockers: nifedipine

Mechanism of action: Nifedipine produces mainly arterial vasodilation by preventing the opening of L-type voltage-gated calcium channels in vascular smooth muscle. This restricts calcium entry and inhibits contractions. Nifedipine can be used in angina, while verapamil, which preferentially acts on the heart, is a useful antiarrhythmic.

Side-effects: Calcium channel blockers are negative inotropes and may exacerbate heart failure. Vasodilation causes flushing and headache.

Angiotensin-converting enzyme (ACE) inhibitors: enalapril

Mechanism of action: Renin is released from the kidneys partly in response to low blood volume. Renin catalyses synthesis of angiotensin I which is then converted to angiotensin II by angiotensin-converting enzyme (ACE). Angiotensin II is a powerful vasoconstrictor and promotes aldosterone release. This causes sodium and water retention. ACE inhibitors prevent angiotensin II formation. They also inhibit the enzymatic breakdown of vasodilator peptides, such as bradykinin, and thereby prolong their action. ACE inhibitors are also used in heart failure.

Side-effects: A test dose of ACE inhibitors must be administered to patients who are in heart failure or taking diuretics, as they may experience an extreme fall in blood pressure following the initial dose (due to a sudden fall in angiotensin II levels). ACE inhibitors rarely cause renal damage in adults but they do produce renal damage in the foetus and must not be given in pregnancy. They may cause a dry cough and hyperkalaemia.

Other antihypertensive agents

Some older antihypertensive agents are shown in the table 'Other antihypertensive agents'. These caused numerous side-effects especially postural hypotension, reflex tachycardia and depression. However α-methyldopa is used in pregnancy-induced hypertension.

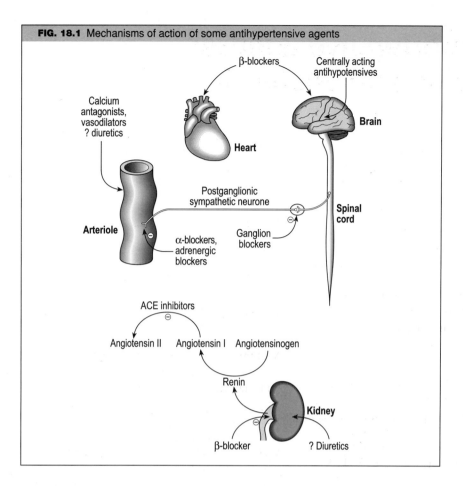

FIG. 18.1 Mechanisms of action of some antihypertensive agents

Other antihypertensive agents

Class	Mechanism of action
Centrally acting agents	
α-Methyldopa	Replaces noradrenaline with α_2-adrenoceptor agonist, α-methylnoradrenaline
Clonidine	α_2-adrenoceptor agonist
Reserpine (rauwolfia alkaloid)	Depletes noradrenaline by inhibiting reuptake into presynaptic vesicles
Ganglion blocker, trimetaphan	Nicotinic antagonist at ganglia
Adrenergic blocking agents, e.g. guanethidine	Deplete and prevent release of noradrenaline in postganglionic sympathetic neurons
α-Adrenoreceptor blocker, prazosin	α_1-Adrenoreceptor antagonist (blocks vasoconstrictor response to catecholamines)
Directly acting vasodilators	
Diltiazem / Minoxidil	Open ATP-dependent potassium channels in smooth muscle, causing hyperpolarisation
Hydralazine	? Stimulates endothelial nitric oxide formation

Antihypertensive agents

- Hypertension (blood pressure consistently greater than 160/95 mmHg) causes cardiovascular disease, strokes and renal failure

- All antihypertensive drugs ultimately reduce peripheral resistance

- The four most widely used types of antihypertensive are:
    1. β-blockers, e.g. atenolol
    2. diuretics, e.g. bendrofluazide
    3. Calcium channel blockers, e.g. nifedipine
    4. angiotensin-converting enzyme (ACE) inhibitors, e.g. enalapril

- Calcium channel blockers reduce calcium availability in vascular smooth muscle and inhibit contractions

- Calcium channel blockers may cause flushing, headaches and exacerbations of heart failure

- ACE inhibitors prevent formation of angiotensin II (a powerful vasoconstrictor) and prolong the action of vasodilator peptides such as bradykinin

- A test dose of ACE inhibitors must be administered to patients in heart failure as they may experience an extreme fall in blood pressure following the initial dose

- α-Methyldopa is used in pregnancy-induced hypertension, but ACE inhibitors must not be used

19 Heart failure: frusemide

Heart failure occurs when, despite normal venous pressures, the heart is unable to maintain sufficient cardiac output to meet the demands of the body. It is present in 1% of those over 65 years. Many patients gradually develop left ventricular failure due to ischaemic heart disease. This causes an increase in pulmonary venous pressure, exudation of interstitial fluid and pulmonary oedema. This produces breathlessness (dypsnoea) and progressive right ventricular failure (leading to peripheral oedema). Cardiogenic shock is an acute, life-threatening condition in which a low cardiac output cannot maintain vital organs. Intravenous drugs for hypotension and pulmonary oedema are required.

The pre-load is the diastolic filling pressure. For the left ventricle pre-load is equivalent to the pulmonary venous pressure. Pre-load increases in heart failure because impaired cardiac output reduces renal perfusion and activates the renin–angiotensin system causing sodium retention and an increased blood volume particularly in the venous system. Sympathetic activation also causes venoconstriction.

Contractility increases because the failing heart cannot eject all the blood presented to it at a normal venous pressure. This causes an increased diastolic volume and compensatory rise in contractility. Increased pre-load and sympathetic drive also increase contractility.

After-load is the resistance against which the ventricle contracts. For the left ventricle after-load is equivalent to the systemic vascular resistance. After-load rises in heart failure due to vasoconstriction following activation of the sympathetic nervous system and renin–angiotensin system. Sympathetic activation also causes tachycardia.

Drug treatment for heart failure

Drugs relieve symptoms (especially dypsnoea). They reduce myocardial work by reducing pre-load (venous pressure) and after-load (arterial blood pressure). The drugs used in heart failure have been reviewed in other chapters. They include the following.

1. *Diuretics* promote renal sodium excretion and a reduction in blood volume, venous pressures and pre-load. They also cause a vasodilation which reduces after-load. Diuretics reduce interstitial fluid formation and relieve pulmonary and peripheral oedema. Thiazides, loop diuretics or combinations are used, depending on the response. Intravenous loop diuretics, such as frusemide, are used in severe pulmonary oedema which results from acute left ventricular failure.

2. *ACE inhibitors* reduce systemic blood pressure (after-load) and venous pressure (pre-load) partly by reducing catecholamine, angiotensin II and aldosterone levels, and by potentiating vasodilator peptides. They are used as adjuvants to diuretics. They can cause hyperkalaemia if used with potassium-sparing agents. First-dose hypotension is a major risk in patients with heart failure and an initial test dose is often given in hospital. ACE inhibitors prolong survival in heart failure.

3. *Positive inotrope infusions*, e.g. the β_1 agonist, dobutamine, are used in cardiogenic shock. The use of digoxin, which is a mild positive inotrope, is controversial in heart failure unless there is a concurrent supraventricular tachycardia.

4. *Vasodilators*, such as glyceryl trinitrate, reduce pre-load by venodilation and reduce after-load by arterial vasodilation. Tolerance develops, so nitrates are used acutely, for ongoing ischaemia, acute heart failure or when ACE inhibitors are contraindicated.

Examples of drugs used in heart failure

Class	Example	Side-effects/comments
Thiazide diuretic	Bendrofluazide	Hypokalaemia
Loop diuretic	Frusemide	Hypokalaemia
ACE inhibitor	Enalapril	First-dose hypotension
Inotrope infusion	Dobutamine (β_1 agonists)*	Used in cardiogenic shock
Vasodilator	Glyceryl trinitrate infusion	Tolerance develops

* Used with low-dose dopamine infusion to improve renal perfusion

Effect of different vasodilators on arterioles and venuoles

Drug	Arterial dilation	Venous dilation
Calcium channel blockers, e.g. nifedipine	+++	+
Nitrates, e.g. glyceryl trinitrate	+	+++
ACE inhibitors, e.g. enalapril	++	++
Loop diuretics (acute), e.g. frusemide	–	++
Directly acting vasodilators, e.g. hydralazine	+++	–
α_1-Antagonists, e.g. prazosin	+++	+
Opiates, e.g. morphine	+	++

– indicates no effect/minimal effect

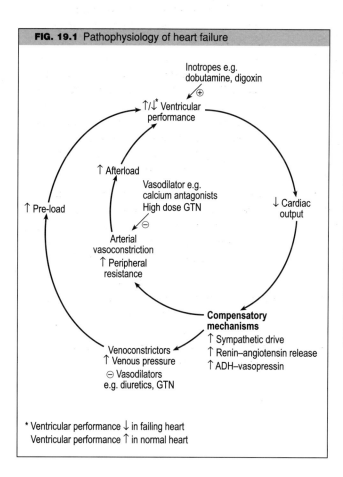

FIG. 19.1 Pathophysiology of heart failure

* Ventricular performance ↓ in failing heart
Ventricular performance ↑ in normal heart

20 Ischaemic heart disease: glyceryl trinitrate and streptokinase

Ischaemic heart disease occurs when the supply of oxygen for myocardial demands is inadequate. This can occur when coronary artery blood flow is impaired by atheroma or spasm. It causes angina (chest pain arising from myocardial ischaemia). Angina is typically exacerbated by exercise and relieved by rest or vasodilator drugs like glyceryl trinitrate. More severe ischaemia (e.g. following coronary artery occlusion by thrombus) produces myocardial death (infarction) or 'heart attacks'. Myocardial infarction (MI) is treated with oxygen, opioid analgesics, aspirin and streptokinase. Cardiac monitoring is essential as MIs can cause sudden lethal arrhythmias. Drugs for angina reduce myocardial work (and therefore oxygen consumption) and increase myocardial oxygen supply by coronary vasodilation. They include β-blockers, calcium channel blockers, vasodilators and fibrinolytics.

β-Blockers and calcium channel blockers:
β-Blockers, such as atenolol, are used in angina because they reduce heart rate and contractility. However, withdrawal may precipitate angina attacks.

Calcium channel blockers, such as nifedipine, reduce contractility and dilate coronary ateries. Arterial dilation reduces after-load. Calcium channel blockers and β-blockers are negative inotropes and may aggravate heart failure.

Vasodilators: glyceryl trinitrate (GTN)

Mechanism of action: Nitrate vasodilators are used to prevent or relieve angina and heart failure. They are converted in endothelial cells into the vasodilator, nitric oxide. This acts on receptors in smooth muscle to cause cyclic GMP synthesis and relaxation. Nitrate vasodilators dilate large veins causing a reduction in venous pressure (pre-load) (see Ch. 19, Heart failure). Larger doses produce arterial dilation and reduce systemic blood pressure (after-load).

Dilation of coronary arterioles increases myocardial blood flow.

Pharmacokinetics: GTN is rapidly metabolised by the liver and is ineffective when swallowed. It is rapidly absorbed through the buccal mucosa when taken sublingually in tablets or as spray. GTN acts very rapidly (in seconds).

Side-effects: Dilation of cerebral and cutaneous arterioles causes headaches and flushing. Postural hypotension and dizziness may occur. GTN has a duration of action of only 20–30 minutes. Longer acting nitrate preparations are available, although tolerance develops to these after several hours. Consequently a nitrate-free period of 4–8 hours is required each day in order that nitrate therapy is effective.

Fibrinolytics: streptokinase

Mechanism of action: Fibrinolytics are enzymes which can dissolve a coronary artery thrombus. This causes reperfusion of the ischaemic tissue around an MI. This will minimise the size of an infarct and reduce the tendency of the ischaemic tissue to produce arrhythmias. Anticoagulant and GTN infusions may also be used acutely.

Aspirin is given with streptokinase. This inhibits platelet aggregation and prevents the arterial clots enlarging. Aspirin is used to prevent MI and strokes.

Pharmacokinetics: Fibrinolytics are given by infusion as soon as possible after an infarct.

Side-effects: Fibrinolytics cause bleeding and are contraindicated following recent trauma, surgery, strokes, peptic ulcers, severe hypertension and other haemorrhagic disorders. Streptokinase is immunogenic and should not be used between 5 days and 12 months of a previous exposure or following any allergic response. Reperfusion can produce arrhythmias.

Nitrate formulations

Nitrate	Administration	Duration of action	Use in angina
GTN or ISDN	Sublingual tablet* or spray	20–30 minutes	Prevention or relief of intermittent episodes
GTN	Transdermal	~12 hours	More frequent attacks
ISMN or ISDN	Modified release tablets	~12 hours	More frequent attacks
GTN or ISDN	Infusion	?	Severe, prolonged angina

GTN, glyceryl trinitrate; ISDN, Isosorbide dinitrate (metabolised to ISMN); ISMN, Isosorbide mononitrate (not subject to first-pass metabolism, so response is more predictable than ISDN)
* GTN tablets have a short shelf-life

Fibrinolytic agents

Fibrinolytic	Indications	Comment
Streptokinase	Myocardial infarction (MI) and other thromboembolic disorders	Co-administered with aspirin. Immunogenic. Cheap. Infused over 1 hour
Tissue plasminogen activator (alteplase)	MI	Co-administered with heparin. Less immunogenic. Expensive
Anistreplase	MI	Immunogenic. Can be given as single i.v. dose (by GP)

REVISION AID
Ischaemic heart disease

- Ischaemic heart disease occurs when the supply of oxygen for myocardial demands is inadequate

- Myocardial ischaemia produces angina (transient chest pain)

- More severe ischaemia produces myocardial infarction (myocardial death) which may cause lethal arrhythmias

- Drugs for angina reduce myocardial work (and therefore oxygen consumption) and increase myocardial oxygen supply by coronary vasodilation. They include β-blockers, calcium channel blockers and vasodilators, such as glyceryl trinitrate (GTN)

- Nitrates cause venodilation and reduce pre-load. Larger doses produce arterial dilation and reduce after-load. Dilation of coronary arterioles increases myocardial blood flow

- Nitrates cause headaches, flushing and exhibit tolerance

- Fibrinolytics, such as streptokinase, dissolve coronary artery thrombus leading to reperfusion of the ischaemic tissue around a myocardial infarction (MI)

- Fibrinolytics cause bleeding and are contraindicated following recent trauma, surgery, strokes, peptic ulcers, severe hypertension and other haemorrhagic disorders

- Streptokinase is immunogenic and should not be used between 5 days and 12 months of a previous exposure, or following any allergic response

- Aspirin inhibits platelet aggregation and prevents the arterial clots enlarging. It is given with streptokinase and is also used to prevent MI and strokes

21 Antiarrhythmic agents: digoxin, atropine and lignocaine

Cardiac arrhythmias (dysrhythmias) are disturbances in the rate or rhythm of the heart contractions. A ventricular rate of less than 60 beats per minute is a bradycardia; a rate of over 100 beats is a tachycardia.

Fibrillations are disorganised muscular contractions which prevent any effective pumping action. Atrial fibrillation (AF) is very common and often asymptomatic although it can precipitate strokes (which can be avoided using anticoagulants), more serious arrhythmias or aggravate heart failure. (In AF the atrial rate may exceed 400 beats per minute but only a proportion of these can be conducted.) By contrast, a myocardial infarction can cause an acute, life-threatening arrhythmia, such as ventricular tachycardia (VT). Patients are breathless, sweating, distressed or unconscious. Ventricular fibrillation (VF) is terminal (it causes cardiac arrest). Electrical cardioversion and intravenous antiarrhythmics are used.

Digoxin

Digoxin (a cardiac glycoside) is used to treat atrial fibrillation with rapid atrioventricular conduction ('fast AF'). This is one kind of supraventricular tachycardia (SVT).

Mechanism of action: Digoxin activates the parasympathetic supply to the heart, via the vagus nerve, by an effect on the central nervous system. This parasympathetic discharge activates muscarinic receptors on cells in the atrioventricular node, causing an increase in potassium conductance, hyperpolarisation and an increase in their refractory period. This slows conductance and reduces the proportion of atrial beats which reach the ventricles.

Digoxin also inhibits the sodium–potassium ATPase on ventricular muscle, causing a small increase in intracellular sodium concentrations. This also leads to a small depolarisation (the pump exchanges $3Na^+$ for $2K^+$). Intracellular sodium inhibits the sodium–calcium antiport system, causing an increase in intracellular calcium and a small increase in cardiac contractility. This may be useful in heart failure.

Pharmacokinetics: Digoxin has a long half-life (~1.5 days) so loading doses are often given to produce a more rapid therapeutic response.

Side-effects: Digoxin can cause many arrhythmias itself, depolarising cells of the conducting system directly and by its sympathomimetic actions. Hypokalaemia predisposes to these arrhythmias. Digoxin, and the diuretics which are often used concurrently, promote potassium excretion. Hence routine monitoring of renal function (digoxin is eliminated by the kidneys), serum potassium and digoxin levels is necessary. Other side-effects include visual disturbances, anorexia, nausea and vomiting.

Atropine and lignocaine

Atropine: This is used to treat bradycardias acutely. These arise due to an infarct affecting the conducting system (called 'heart block'), fibrosis of the atrioventricular node, hypoxia or anaesthesia. Atropine is a muscarinic antagonist which blocks the parasympathetic outflow to the heart that normally slows the heart. Pacemakers are used for persistent bradycardias.

Lignocaine: This is given intravenously in acute ventricular arrhythmias such as VT. Lignocaine, and other class I antiarrhythmics, produce use-dependent block of voltage-operated sodium channels and also delay recovery from their inactivated state (see Ch. 32, Local anaesthetics). This prolongs the absolute refractory period of ventricular muscle, especially in those cells around an infarct from where the arrhythmia may be generated (the 'ectopic focus').

The classification of antiarrhythmic drugs

The Vaughan Williams classification (see table) is based entirely on the electrophysiological responses of ventricular muscle cells. Many antiarrhythmics exert their therapeutic effects on conducting tissue and not on ventricular muscle. However if an arrhythmia is unresponsive to one class of antiarrhythmic then an agent from another class is used. The original classification omits digoxin, atropine and adenosine. (Adenosine opens potassium channels. It is short-acting and can be used as an infusion in SVTs as an alternative to calcium channel blockers. However, unlike calcium channel blockers, adenosine is much less hazardous if accidentally administered in ventricular tachycardia.)

These antiarrhythmics are all negative inotropes and may exacerbate heart failure particularly when they are used in combinations. In particular, intravenous verapamil must never be given to patients receiving β-blockers in any form.

Figure 21.1 shows an alternative classification based on the site of action of antiarrhythmics.

Intravenous adrenaline is given following cardiac arrest. Although adrenaline is actually arrhythmogenic it is used to vasoconstrict peripheral tissues and direct any cardiac output, which might be achieved by cardiac massage, to the heart and brain. Adrenaline is also a positive inotrope.

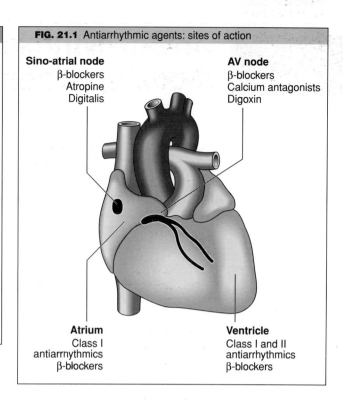

FIG. 21.1 Antiarrhythmic agents: sites of action

Sino-atrial node
β-blockers
Atropine
Digitalis

AV node
β-blockers
Calcium antagonists
Digoxin

Atrium
Class I
antiarrnythmics
β-blockers

Ventricle
Class I and II
antiarrhythmics
β-blockers

The Vaughan Williams classification of antiarrhythmics

Class and example	Site of action	Mechanism
Ia; quinidine	Ventricular muscle	Delays reactivation of sodium channels
Ib; lignocaine	Ventricular muscle	As Ia
Ic; flecainide	Ventricular muscle	As Ia
II; β-blockers, e.g. propranolol	Nodal tissues	Block the arrhythmogenic actions of catecholamines
III; amiodarone (N.B. side-effects include arrhythmias, thyroid disorders and pulmonary fibrosis)	Uncertain (prolongs action potential)	Prolongs action potential by blocking potassium channels (delays repolarisation). Also has class II and IV activity
IV; calcium channel blockers, e.g. verapamil	Nodal tissues	Prevents calcium channel opening to slow conduction and prolongs refractoriness of nodal tissues*

* In nodal tissue calcium influx, not sodium, produces the initial depolarisation of an action potential

Antiarrhythmic agents

- Cardiac arrhythmias (dysrhythmias) are disturbances in the rate or rhythm of heart contractions

- Life-threatening arrhythmias, like ventricular fibrillation, may follow a myocardial infarction and require intravenous drugs

- Other arrhythmias, such as atrial fibrillation, produce few symptoms although they can precipitate strokes (which can be avoided using anticoagulants) or aggravate heart failure

- Digoxin is used to treat atrial fibrillation with rapid atrioventricular conduction ('fast AF'). This is one kind of supraventricular tachycardia

- Digoxin activates the parasympathetic supply to the heart by an undetermined central effect. This reduces the proportion of atrial beats which reach the ventricles

- Digoxin also inhibits the sodium–potassium ATPase transporter on cardiac muscle to produce a small positive inotropic effect

- Digoxin can cause arrhythmias by a direct action on nodal tissues and by its sympathomimetic activity. Hypokalaemia predisposes to these arrhythmias

- Digoxin has a narrow therapeutic index and routine monitoring of renal function, serum potassium and digoxin levels is necessary

- Atropine, a muscarinic antagonist, is used to treat bradycardias

- Lignocaine is given intravenously in ventricular tachycardias

- Lignocaine delays recovery of sodium channels from their inactivated state following repolarisation, and thereby prolongs the refractory period of ventricular muscle cells

- Verapamil must never be given to patients receiving β-blockers

22 Lipid-lowering drugs: cholestyramine

Atherosclerosis is the deposition of fatty material (atheroma) in the walls of medium and large arteries thereby reducing their internal diameter. Atherosclerosis causes ischaemic heart disease, strokes, peripheral vascular disease and renal failure. Smoking, hypertension and high serum lipid levels (especially cholesterol) promote atherosclerosis. Drug treatment is used for cholesterol levels above 6 mM if dietary modification has proven inadequate, although the effect on overall mortality may be small.

Cholesterol is poorly soluble and is transported in the blood with special proteins in small globules termed lipoproteins. Low density lipoprotein (LDL) is the most damaging form of cholesterol while high density lipoprotein (HDL) provides protection against atherosclerosis. Cholesterol can be synthesised de novo or extracted from serum LDLs. It is a precursor of bile acids, steroid hormones and other essential metabolites.

Anion-exchange resins: cholestyramine

These bind bile acids in the intestines and prevent their reabsorption. This promotes the conversion of cholesterol into bile acids by the liver. LDLs are extracted from the plasma to provide the cholesterol. The resins are not absorbed systemically.

Pharmacokinetics: The resins are provided in sachets which should be mixed with water or orange juice. The resins bind other drugs and prevent their absorption. Other drugs should be taken at least 1 hour before or 4–6 hours after cholestyramine.

Side-effects: Gastrointestinal disturbances are common, such as nausea, vomiting, constipation or diarrhoea, heartburn, flatulence and sensations of abdominal bloating.

Other lipid-lowering drugs

Fibrates: bezafibrate: Fibrates stimulate lipoprotein lipase which converts very low density lipoproteins (VLDLs) to LDLs. They also accelerate the clearance of LDLs from the circulation by the liver and increase HDL concentrations.

Side-effects: Fibrates cause gastrointestinal disturbances. Their use is avoided in patients with liver or gallbladder disease as they promote gallstones. They are also avoided for patients who are alcoholic or have renal impairment, as fibrates can cause myositis (inflammation of skeletal muscle which can produce renal damage).

Nicotinic acid (niacin): This vitamin inhibits production of VLDLs leading to a reduction in LDL and total cholesterol concentrations. (VLDLs are precursors of LDL.) Nicotinic acid increases HDL concentrations by inhibiting HDL breakdown.

Side-effects: Flushing, palpitations and gastrointestinal disturbances may limit the use of nicotinic acid although tolerance develops to these side-effects.

HMG-CoA reductase inhibitors: simvastatin: Hydroxy-methyl-glutaryl-coenzyme A reductase catalyses the rate-limiting step for de novo synthesis of cholesterol. Inhibition of this enzyme prevents endogenous cholesterol synthesis, causing an increase in the expression of LDL receptors and removal of LDLs from the circulation.

Side-effects: Myositis occasionally develops. Hence the drugs should be stopped if muscle pains develop.

Fish oil extracts: Their mechanism of action is uncertain. Although they reduce serum triglycerides, they increase serum cholesterol levels. Consequently fish oils are reserved for hypertriglyceridaemias. They may aggravate hypercholesterolaemia.

Side-effects: They produce an unpleasant smell and gastrointestinal disturbances.

Chylomicrons transport absorbed triglycerides from the intestine to the tissues. Very low density lipoproteins (VLDLs) transport endogenously synthesised triglycerides from liver to periphery. Both are hydrolysed in the plasma by lipoprotein lipase. Chylomicrons are converted to chylomicron remnants which are taken up by the liver while VLDLs are converted to low density lipoprotein (LDL). LDL is taken up by the liver and periphery, via high-affinity receptors, in order to provide cellular cholesterol esters. These esters are either transferred to the liver or converted to LDL or VLDL.

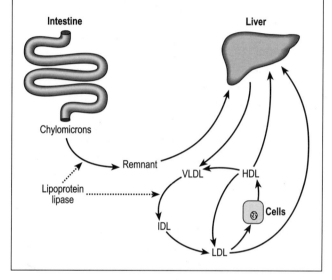

Lipid-lowering drugs

- Atherosclerosis is the deposition of fatty material (atheroma) in the walls of medium and large arteries. This leads to ischaemic heart disease

- Atherosclerosis is accelerated by smoking, hypertension and hyperlipidaemias (especially high levels of LDL cholesterol)

- Anion-exchange resins such as cholestyramine prevent reabsorption of bile acids and promote their synthesis from LDL cholesterol and other sources. They also bind other drugs and prevent their absorption

- Anion-exchange resins and many lipid-lowering drugs cause gastrointestinal disturbances

- Fibrates accelerate the metabolism and extraction of VLDLs and LDLs and increase serum HDL concentrations. They cause gallstones

- Nicotinic acid, and its derivatives, inhibit production of VLDL and therefore reduce LDL and total cholesterol concentrations. They inhibit HDL breakdown. Side-effects limit their use

- HMG-CoA reductase inhibitors prevent de novo synthesis of cholesterol and promote its extraction from plasma LDLs

- Fibrates and HMG-CoA reductase inhibitors can cause myositis

Cholesterol lowering drugs: are they worth it?

Whilst there is a well known relationship between high cholesterol levels and coronary heart disease, the use of lipid lowering drugs is often unnecessary. Although their use correlates with a reduced mortality from coronary heart disease, there is no change in overall mortality. Remarkably, treatment with cholesterol lowering drugs increases death from accidental causes (accidents, suicide or violence). The reason for this association is not known. Consequently treatment with lipid lowering drugs must be used with caution. For a full review of cholesterol lowering drug trials see Muldoon et al 1990 British Medical Journal vol 301: 309–314.

23 Antipsychotics and schizophrenia: haloperidol

Antipsychotic ('neuroleptic') drugs are used to treat psychotic* disorders including mania* and reactions to illicit drugs. However schizophrenia* is the commonest chronic psychotic disorder (affecting 0.5–1% of the population). It places major demands on the NHS because it typically affects young people and has a relapsing and progressive course.

Aetiology: Overactivity of dopamine in the mesolimbic system is widely thought to produce schizophrenia although there is no definitive proof. Evidence for this dopamine hypothesis of schizophrenia includes the facts that all antipsychotic drugs are dopamine antagonists; amphetamine potentiates dopaminergic transmission and can produce a schizophrenia-like state, and dopamine (D_4) receptor density may be found at postmortem to be increased in schizophrenics.

Mechanism of action: Traditional antipsychotic drugs, like haloperidol, are dopamine antagonists. They relieve symptoms in 75% of schizophrenics although improvement is typically partial and the disease often progresses despite medication. Positive symptoms* are improved more than negative* ones. The sedating and anxiolytic effects often produce rapid improvements in disruptive patients. However the true antipsychotic effects (relief of delusions and hallucinations) may take 6 weeks to emerge. Maintenance treatment halves the relapse rate.

Pharmacokinetics: Antipsychotics can be given orally or intramuscularly, particularly if patients are very agitated. Compliance with long-term medication is often poor and slow-release intramuscular depots are widely used, e.g. haloperidol decanoate dissolved in oil.

Side-effects: Movement disorders or 'extrapyramidal effects' are most common with traditional antipsychotics (D_2 receptor antagonists). Acute dystonias (abnormal postures and muscle spasms) and parkinsonism are treated with muscarinic antagonists, e.g. procyclidine. Tardive dyskinesia may develop after several months of treatment, producing jerky or writhing movements. It occurs in 25% of patients taking long-term antipsychotic medication and may be disabling. There is no treatment for established tardive dyskinesia, which may be irreversible.

Akathisia is a subjective feeling of restlessness and compulsion to move. It can be relieved by reducing the dose of antipsychotic or using other anxiolytic drugs. Dopamine antagonists also stimulate prolactin release causing galactorrhoea and infertility.

Neuroleptic malignant syndrome is a potentially fatal acute reaction, particularly in young adults, producing fever, muscular rigidity, delirium and fluctuating blood pressure and heart rate. This is an acute medical emergency. Further use of implicated drugs is contraindicated.

Traditional antipsychotics often produce nondopaminergic side-effects. These include antimuscarinic effects (dry mouth, blurred vision, constipation, urinary retention, confusion and tachycardia); antihistaminic effects (sedation), and anti-alpha adrenergic effects (postural hypotension). Hypothermia, weight gain and depression are also common side-effects.

The vague term 'atypical antipsychotics' refers to many new agents which are relatively free from extrapyramidal effects. Some antagonise dopamine D_4 or 5-HT$_2$ receptors in addition to D_2 receptors.

---

* These terms are explained in the Glossary of psychiatric terms.

Glossary of psychiatric terms

Delusions Fixed false beliefs which are inconsistent with a person's cultural and religious background and persist in spite of overwhelming evidence to the contrary

Functional disorder Disorder with no defect of anatomy, biochemistry or physiology demonstrable using routine clinical investigations

Hallucinations Perceptions without any sensory stimuli

Lack of insight The patient does not realise there is anything wrong with him

Mania A mood disorder typically characterised by euphoria, expansiveness, delusions of grandeur and overactivity. Mania typically alternates with depression

Negative symptoms of schizophrenia. These include apathy, inefficiency, social withdrawal, poverty of speech, flattening of mood and intellectual deterioration

Positive symptoms of schizophrenia. These include hallucinations and delusions

Psychosis A functional disorder (q.v.) characterised by hallucinations (q.v.), delusions (q.v.) and lack of insight (q.v.)

Schizophrenia A psychotic disorder characterised by Schneider's first-rank symptoms such as delusions, auditory hallucination, thought insertion, withdrawal and broadcasting

Other antipsychotic drugs

Antipsychotic drug	Comment/side-effects
Traditional	
Chlorpromazine	Photosensitivity, jaundice, hypothermia
Thioridazine	Fewer movement disorders
Trifluoperazine	Less sedating
Droperidol	Very sedating, useful in mania/aggression
Flupenthixol	Depot widely used
Atypical	
Clozapine	$5\text{-}HT_2$- and D_4-selective antagonist. Causes serious blood dyscrasia
Sulpiride	D_2-selective antagonist
Respiridone	$5\text{-}HT_2$ and D_2 antagonist

REVISION AID

Antipsychotics and schizophrenia

- Antipsychotic ('neuroleptic') drugs are used to treat psychotic disorders including schizophrenia and mania

- Traditional antipsychotic drugs, like haloperidol, are dopamine antagonists

- True antipsychotic effects may take 6 weeks to emerge although sedation may produce a rapid improvement in a patient's behaviour

- Compliance with long-term medication is often poor, and slow-release intramuscular depots are widely used

- Dopaminergic side-effects include akathisia (restlessness), dystonias and parkinsonism. These extrapyramidal effects may respond to antimuscarinic drugs

- Other antipsychotic side-effects include tardive dyskinesia and neuroleptic malignant syndrome

- Other side-effects include: antimuscarinic effects (dry mouth, blurred vision, constipation, urinary retention, confusion and tachycardia); antihistaminic effects (sedation), and anti-alpha adrenergic effects (postural hypotension)

- 'Atypical' antipsychotics may produce fewer extrapyramidal effects

24 Antidepressant drugs: fluoxetine

Monoamine reuptake inhibitors

Depression is characterised by persistent low mood for at least 2 weeks with feelings of hopelessness, helplessness, worthlessness and lack of enjoyment. This typically persists for 3–12 months. There may be anxiety, lack of drive (psychomotor retardation) and even psychotic episodes. 'Biological features' include loss of appetite and weight, early morning waking and poor concentration. The lifetime risk of major depressive illness is around 6%.

Aetiology: Many antidepressant drugs prevent monoamine reuptake or breakdown. This has led to the monoamine hypothesis of depression, which suggests that depression results from an imbalance in the function of the monoamine neurotransmitters noradrenaline, 5HT and dopamine. For the evidence relating to this, see the table 'Arguments for and against monoamine hypothesis of depression'. There is downregulation of β and α_2-adrenergic and 5-HT receptors during chronic antidepressant treatment with a latency similar to the therapeutic response. This is probably more important than the immediate effects of antidepressants therapeutically.

Mechanism of action: The older, tricyclic antidepressants prevent the presynaptic reuptake of noradrenaline and 5-HT (serotonin) and thereby potentiate the effects of these neurotransmitters. Fluoxetine (Prozac) is a serotonin-selective reuptake inhibitor (SSRI). These drugs may take 6 weeks to produce a full therapeutic response.

Pharmacokinetics: Antidepressants are taken orally. Tricyclics enhance the activity of liver enzymes. Sedating antidepressants are usually taken at night.

Side-effects: Tricyclic antidepressants have antimuscarinic effects such as dry mouth, blurred vision, urinary retention, constipation and confusion, although tolerance usually develops to these effects. Sedation is common with the older tricyclics: this may be useful in agitated patients or to assist sleep. Tricyclics

cause weight gain and, in elderly patients, postural hypotension and hyponatraemia. Antidepressants are commonly taken in attempted suicide and may produce cardiac arrhythmias or convulsions. Hence they should be prescribed in small quantities initially. The newer (and more expensive) SSRIs are less sedating and have fewer antimuscarinic and cardiotoxic side-effects.

Monoamine oxidase inhibitors (MAOIs)

These are irreversible, unselective MAO inhibitors (selective, reversible MAO_A inhibitors have recently been developed). They prevent monoamine breakdown. They have serious drug interactions, e.g. extreme hypertension following ingestion of foods such as cheese or drugs such as tricyclic antidepressants.

Manic-depressive psychosis and lithium

Manic-depressive psychosis (bipolar affective disorder) involves alternation between depression and mania typically over a 6-month period. This is 100-fold less common than unipolar depression. Antidepressants and antipsychotics are used during acute episodes; lithium is used prophylactically.

Mechanism of action: This is uncertain. Lithium inhibits breakdown of inositol phosphates and inhibits cAMP production. It affects many neurotransmitters.

Side-effects: Lithium has a low therapeutic index and measurements of serum lithium levels are used to guide treatment and identify toxicity. Renal function must be monitored during treatment as lithium is eliminated by the kidneys. Lithium may impair thyroid and renal function. Acute toxicity can produce nausea, vomiting, thirst, coarse tremor, polyuria and peripheral oedema. Severe intoxication causes psychotic features, coma and convulsions. Rebound mania may occur after lithium treatment is stopped.

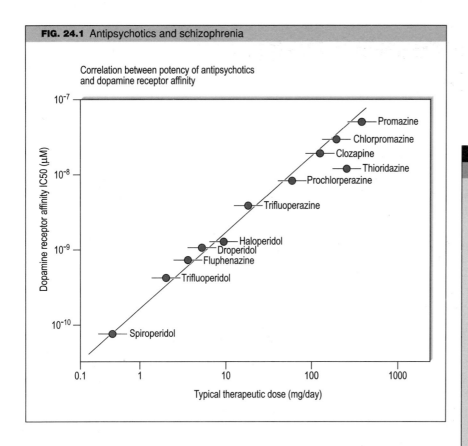

FIG. 24.1 Antipsychotics and schizophrenia

Correlation between potency of antipsychotics and dopamine receptor affinity

Examples of antidepressant drugs

Drug	Uses/comment
SSRIs:	
Fluoxetine, sertraline	Gastrointestinal disturbances
Tricyclics	
Amitriptyline	Sedating
Clomipramine	Obsessive-compulsive disorder
Dothiepin	Sedating
Lofepramine	Useful against psychomotor retardation
Monoamine oxidase inhibitors (MAOIs)	
Phenelzine	Phobias
Moclobemide	Selective, reversible MAO_A inhibitor

Arguments for and against monoamine hypothesis of depression

For	Against
Clinically useful antidepressants enhance monoamine function rapidly	Antidepressants have a delayed therapeutic action (4–6 weeks) but immediate effects on monoamine function
	Other drugs enhance monoamine functions comparably but are not useful antidepressants (e.g. amphetamine)
	Some clinical antidepressants have no effect on transmission by monoamines
Increased 5-HT and dopamine metabolites in cerebrospinal fluid (CSF) of depressed patients	The same biochemical changes as in depression often occur in mania
There is monoamine regulation of some pituitary responses which are impaired in depression	

25 Sedatives, anxiolytics and hypnotics: temazepam

A sedative is a drug which tends to calm, moderate or 'tranquillize' nervousness or excitement. Anxiolytic drugs are used to treat anxiety, i.e. a feeling of apprehension and unease over an impending or anticipated ill. Hypnotics are drugs used to enhance the initiation or maintenance of sleep. Of the UK population, 17% use anxiolytic drugs regularly.

Mechanism of action: All anxiolytics and hypnotics are sedatives. Benzodiazepines are the commonest sedatives in use. They increase the affinity of $GABA_A$ receptors for GABA and thereby enhance its actions. (GABA is the commonest inhibitory neurotransmitter in the brain.) Benzodiazepines are not GABA agonists as they bind to a separate site on the $GABA_A$ receptor. No endogenous agonist at the benzodiazepine binding site has been discovered so far.

Benzodiazepines and the $GABA_B$ agonist, baclofen, are centrally acting muscle relaxants. They are used to relieve the muscle spasticity associated with spinal injuries, and benzodiazepines are used to treat epilepsy.

The benzodiazepines are often used as sedatives in combination with antipsychotics during acute psychosis, particularly if patients are aggressive or very agitated.

Pharmacokinetics: Benzodiazepines are metabolised in the liver. They have many active metabolites which prolong their action. Long-acting benzodiazepines (e.g. diazepam) are traditionally used as anxiolytics because they will have an effect through the day, and they are also used in alcohol detoxification regimes. Short-acting benzodiazepines,

such as temazepam, are used as hypnotics and premeds (anxiolytics given prior to surgery).

Side-effects: Benzodiazepine dependence has now been identified as a major problem (see Ch. 26, Drug misuse and dependence). Hence prescription of many benzodiazepines is now limited to specialists. They should be prescribed in short courses (less than 2 weeks). Antipsychotic drugs can be used temporarily as alternatives in severe anxiety states (e.g. withdrawal syndromes).

Benzodiazepines should not be used for the treatment of depression, phobias, obsessive-compulsive disorders and psychoses, as there are better alternatives; most benzodiazepines have no antidepressant or antipsychotic actions.

Benzodiazepines are commonly taken in suicide attempts although they are seldom lethal except in very large quantities or following injection. (Benzodiazepines have replaced barbiturates as sedatives/hypnotics. Barbiturate overdose is far more dangerous and they are more addictive than benzodiazepines.)

Other side-effects include: respiratory depression, although this is usually insignificant except in severe respiratory disorders, disinhibition, which may produce aggression, and rebound anxiety or insomnia upon withdrawal.

All sedatives tend to impair the speed and accuracy of mental processes. This may affect driving or performance at work or produce confusion in the elderly.

FIG. 25.1 Metabolism of benzodiazepines

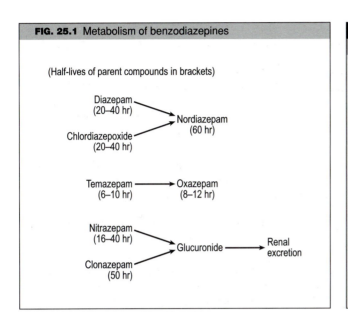

(Half-lives of parent compounds in brackets)

Diazepam (20–40 hr) → Nordiazepam (60 hr)
Chlordiazepoxide (20–40 hr) → Nordiazepam (60 hr)

Temazepam (6–10 hr) → Oxazepam (8–12 hr)

Nitrazepam (16–40 hr) → Glucuronide → Renal excretion
Clonazepam (50 hr) → Glucuronide → Renal excretion

REVISION AID

Sedatives, anxiolytics and hypnotics

- Benzodiazepines increase the affinity of the $GABA_A$ receptor for the inhibitory neurotransmitter, GABA

- Benzodiazepines are not GABA agonists as they bind to a separate site on the $GABA_A$ receptor

- Benzodiazepines have many active metabolites which prolong their action

- Short-acting benzodiazepines, such as temazepam, are used as hypnotics and premeds

- Long-acting benzodiazepines are traditionally used as anxiolytics

- Benzodiazepine dependence is a major problem. They should be prescribed in short courses (less than 2 weeks)

- Sedatives may produce confusion in the elderly or exacerbate respiratory diseases

Sedatives and related drugs

Drug	Use
Benzodiazepines	
Temazepam	Premed, hypnotic
Diazepam (Valium)	Anxiolytic
Diazemuls (intravenous diazepam)	Sedative for surgery or status epilepticus
Nitrazepam	Hypnotic
Chlordiazepoxide (Librium)	Detoxification regimes
Clonazepam	Antiepileptic
Nonbenzodiazepines	
Zopiclone	Hypnotic
Buspirone (5-HT$_{1A}$ agonist)	Anxiolytic (metabolite is α_2 agonist)
Chloral hydrate	Hypnotic (repeated use causes headache)
Chlormethiazole (Heminevrin)	Detoxification regimes (addictive)

26 Drug misuse and dependence

Drug misuse is drug-taking which is hazardous or harmful and unsanctioned by professional or cultural standards. Drug dependence (addiction) is a state resulting from repeated administration of a drug, characterised by a compulsion to take the drug continually or periodically, and sometimes to avoid the discomfort of its absence (a withdrawal syndrome). Not all drug misusers are drug-dependent. Nicotine and alcohol addiction are considered in a separate chapter.

Aetiology: Drug misuse is initiated and maintained for several reasons:

1. drugs confer pleasurable effects (this is greatly influenced by the setting and expectation of the user);
2. social pressure, tolerance and encouragement (especially with regard to alcohol);
3. availability;
4. self-medication to relieve withdrawal syndromes, social phobia or the pain of unsatisfactory relationships;
5. personal factors, e.g. curiosity or boredom.

There is no single physiological explanation for drug dependence. However many drugs promote release of dopamine from a pathway from the ventral tegmental area to the nucleus accumbens. This 'reward' pathway is activated by opioids, alcohol and nicotine.

Classification: There are five categories of abused drugs (see the table 'Classification of misused drugs').

1. *Opioids* (e.g. diamorphine or heroin) produce euphoria (a feeling of wellbeing). Withdrawal is usually preceded by substitution with oral methadone elixir. This has a longer half-life than heroin, avoids the need to buy and to inject diamorphine and produces less severe withdrawal symptoms.

2. *Sedatives* produce sleep, relief from anxiety and social and sexual disinihibition.

3. *Stimulants* elevate mood, increase wakefulness, give an enhanced sense of mental and physical energy. Cocaine is highly addictive when the volatile compound ('crack' or 'free base') is sniffed. Dependence causes drastic

personal and social disruption. Withdrawal from stimulants may cause insomnia and depression but has few physical effects.

4. *Hallucinogens* produce multiple strange, intense effects including hallucinations. The acute effects of these drugs put users at risk of accidents and suicide.

5. *Miscellaneous* classes. Cannabis is a sedative and hallucinogen, although its toxicity is low. However cannabis may be a 'gateway' drug, giving access to other illicit drugs. Solvents (glue, lighter fuels) produce sedation and hallucinations. Intoxication may produce suffocation or pulmonary aspiration, and users are often adolescents.

Methods of administration: Combinations of drugs are often used (e.g. heroin with cocaine). Most drug addicts also smoke tobacco. Oral administration carries the lowest hazards, although effects are slower in onset and less intense; larger doses are required making oral administration less 'cost-efficient'. Smoking, chewing, inhalation and sniffing allow absorption through the nasal mucosa and lungs. This avoids first-pass metabolism producing more rapid and intense effects. Intravenous injection produces the most intense effects and requires the least quantity of drug. However it carries the greatest risks, including overdose, dependence and infection.

Management: Management involves minimising the hazards of drug misuse, provision of withdrawal or substitute medication and attention to the social and psychological problems which maintain drug misuse. Withdrawal must often be repeated several times to achieve complete abstinence. However many users of illicit drugs spontaneously progress onto alcohol and tobacco by middle age.

Many addictive drugs produce psychological withdrawal syndromes or craving, i.e. an overpowering desire for the administration of the drug. Abrupt discontinuation is usually possible unless there is a physical withdrawal syndome. (See table 'Features of physical withdrawal syndromes'.)

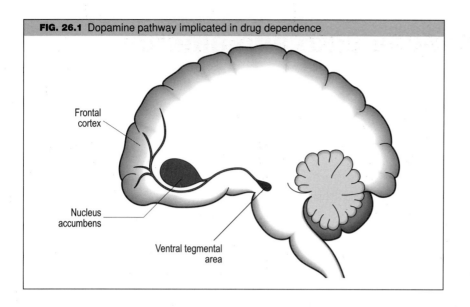

FIG. 26.1 Dopamine pathway implicated in drug dependence

Frontal cortex

Nucleus accumbens

Ventral tegmental area

Classification of misused drugs

Class	Examples	Route	Dependence potential	Drug-specific side-effects
Opioids	Heroin	Injected (or smoked)	Very high	Respiratory arrest
Stimulants	Cocaine (crack)	Sniffed	Very high	Disturbed behaviour
	Amphetamine	Oral (or injected)	Moderate	Psychosis
	Ecstasy*	Oral	"	"
Benzodiazepine sedatives	Diazepam	Oral	High	Withdrawal seizures
	Temazepam	Oral (or injected)	"	"
Hallucinogen	LSD	Oral	Low	Disturbed behaviour
Sedative/hallucinogen	Cannabis†	Smoked	Low	? Psychosis
	Solvents	Inhaled	Low	Suffocation, aspiration
Stimulant/sedative	Nicotine	Smoked (or chewed)	Very high	See Ch. 27
Sedative	Alcohol	Oral	High	See Ch. 27

* Ecstasy is methylene dioxymethamphetamine (MDMA)
† The active metabolite in cannabis is tetrahydrocannabinol (THC)

Features of physical withdrawal syndromes

Opioids	Benzodiazepines
Nausea, vomiting, diarrhoea	Anxiety symptoms: anxiety, sweating, insomnia, headache, shaking, nausea
Restlessness anxiety, irritability, sleeplessness	Disordered perceptions: feeling of unreality, abnormal body sensations and hypersensitivity
Pains in muscles, bones and joints	Psychosis
Running nose and eyes, sneezing, sweating	Epileptiform seizures
Dilated pupils, gooseflesh, flushing	
Opioid withdrawal ('cold turkey') resembles the features of a bad cold	Benzodiazepine withdrawal is particularly difficult and may take several months

REVISION AID
Drug misuse and dependence

- Drug misuse is drug taking which is hazardous or harmful and unsanctioned by professional or cultural standards

- Drug dependence (addiction) is a state resulting from repeated administration of a drug, characterised by a compulsion to take the drug continually or periodically, and sometimes to avoid the discomfort of its absence (a withdrawal syndrome)

- Drug misuse is initiated and maintained by multiple pharmacological, psychological and social factors

- Many abused drugs stimulate release of dopamine in a reward pathway in the brain from the ventral tegmental area to the nucleus accumbens

- Abused drugs can be classified as: opioids, sedatives, stimulants and hallucinogens although cannabis, solvents and nicotine cannot easily be classified

- Combinations of drugs are often used, e.g. heroin with cocaine

- Oral administration carries the least hazards although effects are slower in onset and less intense

- Intravenous injection produces the most intense effects and requires the least quantity of drug. However it carries the greatest risks including overdose, dependence and infection

27 Tobacco smoking and alcohol

Smoking

In the UK 30–35% of adults smoke while 1 in 5 people die prematurely from smoking-related diseases.

Effects of smoking (Fig. 27.1): Smoking permits rapid absorption of nicotine, an agonist at nicotinic acetylcholine receptors. This produces excitation of autonomic and central neurons. These responses desensitise at high nicotine concentrations. Nicotine produces vasoconstriction, psychological arousal or sedation, and dependence.

Carcinogens in tobacco smoke include polycyclic hydrocarbons and nitrosamines. Lung cancer has a poor prognosis and 90% of cases are smoking-related. Asbestos exposure further increases the incidence of lung cancer amongst smokers. The incidence of bronchitis, ischaemic heart disease, peptic ulcers and oral, oesophageal and bladder cancer are all increased by smoking.

Smoking produces high levels of carboxyhaemoglobin thereby reducing oxygen transport and exacerbating cardiorespiratory disorders. Smoking also disrupts immunological functions, immobilises respiratory tract cilia and produces foetal growth retardation. Environmental tobacco smoke increases rates of childhood asthma.

Nicotine withdrawal: This produces irritability, aggressiveness, sleep disturbances and impaired mental performance for 2–3 weeks although craving may persist for much longer. Methods to reduce the dangers of smoking (e.g. smoking low tar cigarettes) produce only small benefits. However active encouragement can motivate many smokers to stop.

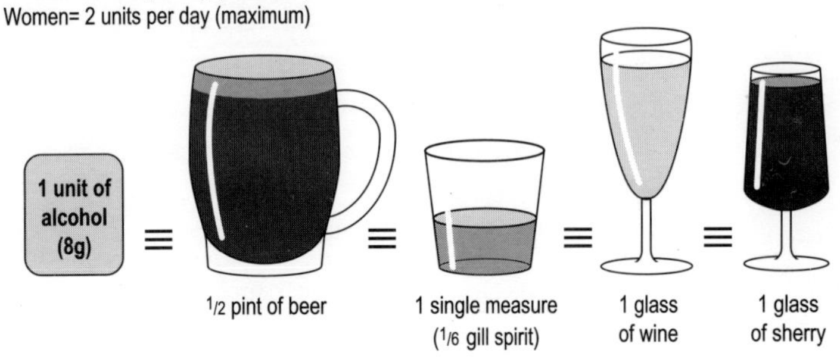

Alcohol

In the population of the UK 2–5% have alcohol-related problems. Alcohol causes about three-quarters of the 2500 deaths from chronic liver disease each year.

Acute effects: Alcohol depresses neuronal activity in a similar manner to that of general anaesthetics producing vasodilation, slurred speech, lack of motor coordination, euphoria and sedation. Physical injury may arise due to disinhibition causing poor judgement, mood changes and recklessness. Hangovers are produced by additional substances in the beverage. Alcohol is a diuretic as it inhibits ADH release.

Chronic effects: These include the following.

1. Gastrointestinal disease including cirrhosis, liver and pancreas disease, peptic ulcers, cancer of the oesophagus and rectum.
2. Brain damage, e.g. Wernicke–Korsakoff syndrome (thiamine deficiency).
3. Miscellanous conditions, e.g. chest infections, Cushing's syndrome (excess glucocorticoid secretion), cardiomyopathies, gout, induction of liver enzymes and foetal abnormalities. Alcoholics often become malnourished, with consequent medical effects.

The combination of acute disinhibition, brain damage and behavioural addiction produces multiple social problems including domestic violence, child abuse, delinquency and suicide. However moderate ethanol consumption may protect against ischaemic heart disease by increasing serum HDL concentrations and inhibiting platelet aggregation.

Alcohol withdrawal: This causes tremor, insomnia, agitation, fits and acute confusion (delirium tremens). This can be avoided using reducing doses of sedative drugs over a week.

Management of alcoholism: This involves acute detoxification and psychological and social support. In aversion therapy the acetaldehyde dehydrogenase inhibitor, disulphiram, is used. This interacts with alcohol causing accumulation of acetaldehyde leading to vomiting, palpitations, flushing, colic and dizziness (a large alcohol intake may be fatal).

FIG. 27.1 Sensible drinking

Sensible drinking
Men= 3 units per day (maximum)
Women= 2 units per day (maximum)

1 unit of alcohol (8g) = ½ pint of beer = 1 single measure (1/6 gill spirit) = 1 glass of wine = 1 glass of sherry

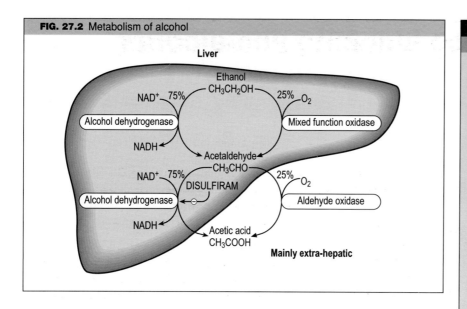

FIG. 27.2 Metabolism of alcohol

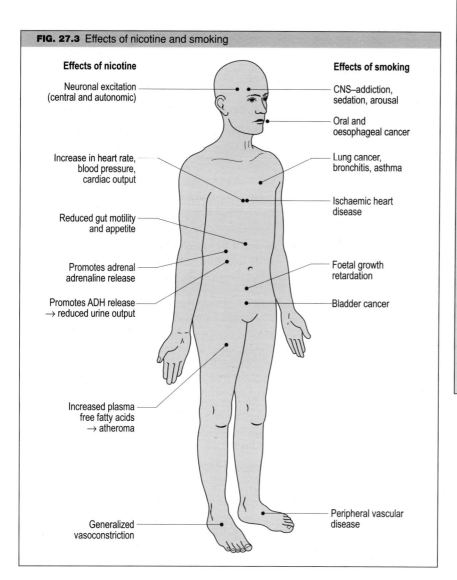

FIG. 27.3 Effects of nicotine and smoking

28 Nonsteroidal antiinflammatory drugs (NSAIDs): aspirin

Nonsteroidal antiinflammatory drugs (NSAIDs) are used:

1. to treat mild pain (*analgesic* action);
2. to treat rheumatoid arthritis (*antiinflammatory* action);
3. to treat pyrexia, i.e. the high temperature of fevers (*antipyretic* action);
4. to prevent myocardial infarctions (*antiplatelet* action).

Mechanism of action: NSAIDs inhibit cyclooxygenase. This prevents the synthesis of prostaglandins, prostacylin and thromboxanes. The therapeutic actions are explained below.

Analgesia: Pain is often caused by an inflammatory response to tissue injury; this might occur at the site of a bruise or a joint sprain. Such inflammatory responses produce local prostaglandins which activate peripheral pain fibres. NSAIDs prevent the synthesis of these prostaglandins and so reduce the pain. They may act directly to prevent conduction of pain impulses in the central nervous system, and thereby relieve pains with no obvious inflammatory mechanism (such as 'tension headaches').

Antiinflammatory action: Rheumatoid arthritis is caused by a persistent inflammation of tissues in the joints. This causes pain and progressively destroys the joints. Prostaglandins are important activators of the immune system and inhibition of their synthesis reduces the inflammatory responses which occur in rheumatoid arthritis.

Antipyretic action: Pyrexia is a feature of infection. This may arise due to the synthesis of prostaglandins in the hypothalamus in response to the release of other substances from the site of infection. NSAIDs prevent the synthesis of prostaglandins and prevent pyrexia.

Antiplatelet action: Platelet aggregation in response to atheroma is thought to initiate the blockage of coronary arteries causing myocardial infarction (heart attack). Platelet aggregation is promoted by thromboxane A. NSAIDs inhibit thromboxane production and thereby prevent platelet aggregation.

Pharmacokinetics: NSAIDs are available in many formulations, including parenteral preparations for patients who cannot drink (such as postoperative patients).

NSAIDs are commonly taken in deliberate self-poisonings (parasuicide). Aspirin is an acidic drug which can form solid boluses in the stomach. Hence gastric lavage (stomach pumping) is effective up to 24 hours after an overdose.

Side-effects: NSAIDs cause peptic ulcers. These produce pain and intestinal bleeding. Peptic ulcers may arise because NSAIDs prevent the synthesis of prostaglandins, which normally inhibit the secretion of gastric acid. Hence NSAIDs (especially aspirin) cause an increase in gastric acidity, and they should be avoided in patients with peptic ulcers or used with an antiulcer drug such as misoprostol.

NSAIDs should be avoided in patients with renal or heart disease as they interfere with blood flow within the kidneys. This can cause renal impairment and fluid retention.

NSAIDs are avoided in pregant women as they may cause closure of the ductus arteriosis.

Other adverse reactions include allergic reactions (especially to aspirin), abdominal discomfort, which may be avoided by taking NSAIDs with food or milk, diarrhoea and anaemia. Aspirin should be avoided in children as it can precipitate Reyes' syndrome.

Other NSAIDs

NSAID	Notes
Paracetamol (nonopioid analgesic)	Antipyretic elixir. No antiinflammatory actions. Causes liver damage in overdose
Ibuprofen, naproxen	Few side-effects; suitable for first-line treatment
Mefenamic acid	Commonly used to treat dysmenorrhoea
Diclofenac, ketorolac	Stronger analgesics but with more side-effects
Indomethacin	Strong analgesic, often used in rheumatoid arthritis
Piroxicam	Strong NSAID, longer half-life so can be taken once daily
Phenylbutazone	Very strong antiinflammatory agent, can produce serious side-effects

FIG. 28.1 Effects of nonsteroidal antiinflammatory drugs (NSAIDs)

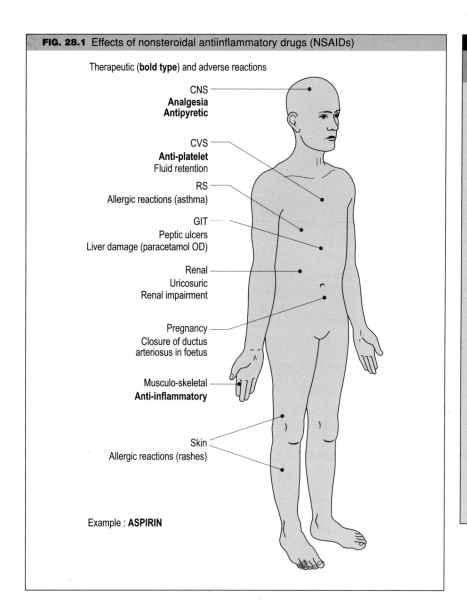

Therapeutic (**bold type**) and adverse reactions

CNS
Analgesia
Antipyretic

CVS
Anti-platelet
Fluid retention

RS
Allergic reactions (asthma)

GIT
Peptic ulcers
Liver damage (paracetamol OD)

Renal
Uricosuric
Renal impairment

Pregnancy
Closure of ductus
arteriosus in foetus

Musculo-skeletal
Anti-inflammatory

Skin
Allergic reactions (rashes)

Example : **ASPIRIN**

REVISION AID

Nonsteroidal antiinflammatory drugs (NSAIDs)

- Mild or moderate pain can be treated using nonsteroidal antiinflammatory drugs (NSAIDs), such as aspirin

- NSAIDs prevent the synthesis of prostaglandins

- NSAIDs are used to treat pain, inflammation (e.g. in rheumatoid arthritis) and pyrexia (fever). NSAIDs are widely used to prevent heart attacks and strokes, because they inhibit platelet aggregation and therefore prevent arterial thrombosis (clots) and infarction (tissue death)

- Gastric ulceration is the most important adverse reaction to NSAIDs. Chronic use of these drugs can produce ulcers which can lead to fatal internal bleeding (GI haemorrhages)

- Paracetamol is related to NSAIDs although it is better considered as a nonopioid analgesic. Paracetamol is the drug most commonly taken in overdose in the UK. It can cause severe liver damage. Paracetamol overdose is treated with acetylcysteine

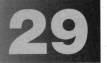

Opioid analgesics: morphine

Opioids are drugs which produce similar actions to morphine and are antagonised by naloxone. They are the most potent analgesics available. (The term 'opiate' refers to any naturally occurring morphine-like drug.)

Mechanism of action: Opioids are agonists at cellular opioid receptors. They produce a decrease in membrane calcium conductance, an increase in potassium conductance and an inhibition of cAMP synthesis. This causes hyperpolarisation of nerve cells making them less excitable. Hence opioids inhibit neuronal functions. Most opioid effects arise from their action at μ-opioid receptors in the central nervous system. Analgesia occurs due to inhibition of substance P release in the substantia gelatinosa of the spinal cord. Also the 5HT systems become more active in the nucleus raphe magnus, the periaqueductal grey and the thalamus.

Pharmacokinetics: Opioids are usually given intramuscularly or intravenously for severe pain. Oral formulations are available for those with chronic severe pain. Morphine is metabolised by the liver to morphine glucuronide. This is excreted by the kidney and into the bile where it undergoes enterohepatic recirculation.

Side-effects: Opioids produce severe respiratory depression by inhibiting the normal response of the central chemoreceptors to high levels of carbon dioxide. The respiratory rate is affected more than the respiratory volume. Hence opioid-induced respiratory depression is characterised by infrequent deep breaths. Naloxone can be used to treat apnoea in acute overdosage.

Opioids exhibit tolerance; the effect of the same dose decreases following repeated administration. Tolerance occurs to the analgesic, euphoric, sedative, respiratory depression and emetic effects of opioids but not to the constipating or miotic effects. Increased doses are required to produce the same analgesic effect (or euphoria in the case of addicts). This is partly due to a reduction in opioid-receptor responsiveness and to increased drug metabolism. However analgesic requirements may also increase as a painful condition, such as cancer, progresses.

Opioid administration produces euphoria: a feeling of contentment and well-being. This has led to the repeated illicit use of opioids, ultimately producing addiction. κ-Opioid receptor agonists may produce unpleasant feelings termed 'dysphoria'. Addiction is characterised by a withdrawal syndrome upon sudden cessation of drug use. This produces extreme craving for the drug and physical symptoms which resemble a bad cold. Addiction rarely develops following the therapeutic use of opioids.

Opioids are usually administered with an antiemetic drug, because nausea and vomiting occurs in 40% of patients after a single dose.

Opioids produce disorganised peristalsis which reduces gut mortality. This causes constipation and delays stomach emptying. Tolerance to this effect does not develop. Hence opioids are usually administered with laxatives. Furthermore, opioids increase smooth muscle tone. This may aggravate biliary and renal colic. These effects occur due to peripheral opioid receptors in the myenteric nerve plexus of the gut.

Miosis (constriction of the pupil) is produced by an effect on the nucleus of the third cranial nerve. Although this rarely disturbs vision it is an important sign of opioid overdose.

The sedating properties of opioids make them useful premeds. They also induce sleep (narcosis) and are therefore known as narcotic analgesics. They suppress the cough reflex and are used as antitussives.

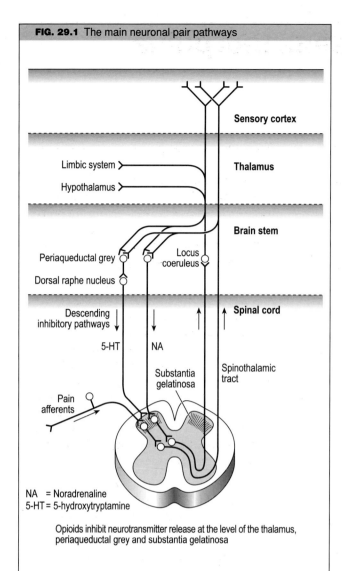

FIG. 29.1 The main neuronal pair pathways

Sensory cortex

Thalamus

Limbic system

Hypothalamus

Brain stem

Periaqueductal grey

Locus coeruleus

Dorsal raphe nucleus

Spinal cord

Descending inhibitory pathways

5-HT   NA

Substantia gelatinosa

Spinothalamic tract

Pain afferents

NA   = Noradrenaline
5-HT = 5-hydroxytryptamine

Opioids inhibit neurotransmitter release at the level of the thalamus, periaqueductal grey and substantia gelatinosa

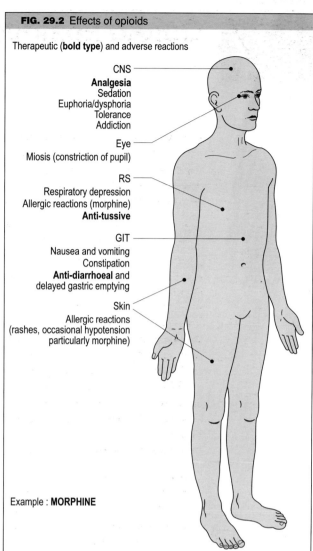

FIG. 29.2 Effects of opioids

Therapeutic (**bold type**) and adverse reactions

CNS
Analgesia
Sedation
Euphoria/dysphoria
Tolerance
Addiction

Eye
Miosis (constriction of pupil)

RS
Respiratory depression
Allergic reactions (morphine)
Anti-tussive

GIT
Nausea and vomiting
Constipation
Anti-diarrhoeal and
delayed gastric emptying

Skin
Allergic reactions
(rashes, occasional hypotension
particularly morphine)

Example : **MORPHINE**

Opioid drugs, their uses and analgesic potencies

Drug	Comment	Analgesic potency compared to morphine
Morphine	May cause histamine release producing hypotension and allergic reactions	1
Diamorphine	Prodrug metabolised to morphine. More lipid-soluble and penetrates CNS faster causing enhanced euphoria	1.5
Codeine	Prodrug metabolised to morphine. More reliable oral absorption. Used as mild analgesic, antitussive and antidiarrhoeal	0.02 (i.e. 1/50th of the potency of morphine)
Pethidine	Used widely in labour, as causes less potent respiratory depression than morphine	0.1 (i.e. 1/10th of the potency of morphine)
Methadone	Prescribed for addicts as an oral substitute for intravenous opioids. Long duration causing less severe withdrawal syndrome	

REVISION AID

Opioid analgesics

- Opioids are drugs which produce similar actions to morphine and are antagonised by naloxone

- They are agonists at opioid receptors and inhibit neuronal function

- They are the strongest analgesics available

- Their principal side-effects are respiratory depression, nausea and vomiting and constipation

- Other effects include euphoria, sedation, tolerance and addiction

- They may be used as antidiarrhoeals and antitussives

- Overdosage produces respiratory arrest and miosis (constriction of the pupil). This can be treated with naloxone

30 General anaesthetics: thiopentone and halothane

Modern anaesthetists practise *balanced anaesthesia*. This involves the use of drugs to achieve three effects: anaesthesia, analgesia and muscle relaxation (see later). General anaesthetics produce complete loss of consciousness and thereby prevent awareness of the pain of surgery. Skeletal muscle paralysis, endotracheal intubation and mechanical ventilation may also be required, for example, to prevent pulmonary aspiration (inhalation of the stomach contents) which can produce fatal chemical pneumonia.

Volatile (gaseous) anaesthetics may take several minutes to produce the level of anaesthesia required for surgery. A period of excitation often occurs during gaseous induction which can lead to aspiration and injury. To avoid this, rapid induction is achieved using short-acting, intravenous anaesthetics. One of the most popular of these induction agents is the barbiturate, thiopentone. After induction anaesthesia is usually maintained using a volatile anaesthetic such as halothane.

Mechanism of action: There is wide controversy in this field but much recent evidence indicates that surgical concentrations of general anaesthetics block synaptic transmission by specifically binding to parts of receptor-operated ion channels. This potentiates inhibitory neurotransmitters, such as GABA, and inhibits excitatory neurotransmitters like glutamate.

General anaesthetics do not disrupt the lipid membrane of cells or influence voltage-operated ion channels at therapeutic concentrations; nor do they inhibit action potential conduction. However these effects can be produced at the very high concentrations achieved in experimental situations.

Pharmacokinetics: Induction agents produce anaesthesia in seconds, i.e. one *arm–brain circulation time*. Their anaesthetic action is terminated by redistribution from nervous tissue (which has a high blood flow but low volume) into tissues with lower blood flows but greater mass (e.g. muscle). Thiopentone persists at subanaesthetic concentrations for many hours in these tissues until it is metabolised by the liver. Hence repeated doses lead to accumulation which delays reversal of anaesthesia and causes residual drowsiness.

Volatile anaesthetic agents, such as halothane, are administered by inhalation. They take longer to produce anaesthesia than intravenous agents but are eliminated more rapidly. Furthermore the plasma concentration responds quickly to changes in the inhaled concentration. This allows rapid readjustment of the depth of anaesthesia during maintenance which cannot be achieved with most intravenous agents. Of the inhaled halothane, 20% is metabolised by the liver. This may contribute to its side-effects.

Side effects: All general anaesthetic agents suppress protective reflexes. This puts patients at risk of aspiration.

General anaesthetics reduce blood pressure. This can produce tissue infarction in those with ischaemic vascular disease or those with pre-existing hypotension following severe haemorrhage. Cardiac arrhythmias are common in anaesthetised patients, partly because of the arrhythmogenic action of agents like halothane, and also in response to surgical manipulation.

Halothane can produce a very rare but serious form of hepatitis, and must not be used repeatedly over short periods. Unfortunately the other volatile agents are irritating to the airways and are less suitable for gaseous induction (particularly in children).

Other induction agents

Drug	Comments
Propofol	Rapid hepatic elimination. Does not accumulate. May be used by infusion to maintain anaesthesia
Etomidate	Minimal cardiovascular system (CVS) depression. Used in patients with CVS disease. Infusions cause adrenal suppression
Ketamine	Blocks ion channel of NMDA (glutamate) receptors. Minimal respiratory and CVS depression. Causes hallucinations

Other volatile anaesthetic agents

Drug	Comments
Isoflurane	Irritant to airways
Enflurane	Irritant to airways. May aggravate epilepsy
Nitrous oxides (gaseous rather than volatile agent)	Low potency. Used as analgesic particularly in 50:50 combination with oxygen (Entonox)

Mechanisms of action for Anaesthetics

Almost a century ago Meyer and Overton proposed that the anaesthetic potency was linked to the lipid solubility (high lipid solubility = high potency). From this a series of theories have been developed to explain the action of anaesthetics.

- *Changes in membrane fluidity.* This theory proposed that anaesthetics inserted themselves into the lipid membrane. This accumulation caused a disruption in the ordering of the lipid bilayer and so affect membrane bound proteins e.g. ion channels.

- *Expansion of membrane volume.* Here accumulation of anaesthetic molecules causes an increase in the volume of the membrane layer. This crowding of the lipid bilayer would then affect any membrane bound protein.

- *Hydrogen bond disruption.* As hydrogen bonding is an essential mechanism in maintaining the structure of many molecules. It may be that anaesthetics can act to disrupt hydrogen bonds in a lipid or protein molecule. Consequently loss of the correct structure could lead to alteration in function.

- *Direct interaction with proteins.* It may be that anaesthetics can directly interact with protein molecules (not necessarily just those in the cell membrane). They could interact with the agonist binding sites on receptors, or a distinct modulatory site, or they could act within the actual ion channel, physically blocking the flow of ions.

Whilst the first two theories have fallen out of favour (as clinical concentrations often have only a minor effect on membrane volume or fluidity) all ultimately result in a change in protein function. It seems unlikely therefore that anaesthetics act to alter the function of many integral proteins, such as ion channels, and it is through these changes that anaesthesia is induced. For a better and more comprehensive discussion see Peoples et al 1996 Annual Review of Pharmacology and Toxicology vol 36: 185–201.

REVISION AID
General anaesthetics

- Balanced anaesthesia requires drugs to produce anaesthesia, analgesia and muscle relaxation

- Induction agents such as thiopentone are rapidly acting, intravenous general anaesthetics which avoid the dangerous period of excitation produced by gaseous induction

- Surgical concentrations of general anaesthetics enhance inhibitory neurotransmitters and diminish the effects of excitatory ones

- The action of induction agents is terminated by redistribution. However these agents may remain in the body for several hours

- Volatile anaesthetic agents, such as halothane, are administered by inhalation which allows rapid elimination and accurate readjustment of the depth of anaesthesia

- General anaesthesia puts patients at risk of pulmonary aspiration. This can be prevented by endotracheal intubation

- General anaesthetics produce hypotension and arrhythmias

31 Neuromuscular blocking agents: suxamethonium and vecuronium

General anaesthetics produce loss of protective reflexes, including the cough reflex. This puts patients at risk of pulmonary aspiration (inhalation of the gastric contents) which can be fatal. It is prevented by sealing off the trachea from the pharynx using a hollow, cuffed, endotracheal tube. Insertion of these tubes into the trachea (intubation) produces violent coughing even in anaesthetised patients. This is prevented by using neuromuscular blocking agents. These produce paralysis of voluntary muscle. This may also permit mechanical ventilation, which is required for many operations, and prevent unconscious movements in response to surgical stimulation. (Involuntary movements may also be prevented using high concentrations of anaesthetic agents. However this is slower in onset and produces side-effects such as hypotension and arrhythmias.)

Mechanism of action: Neuromuscular blocking agents act on the subdivision of nicotinic cholinergic receptors located at the skeletal neuromuscular junction. Surprisingly both agonists and antagonists of these receptors produce paralysis.

Agonists at these receptors are known as depolarising neuromuscular blocking agents. Suxamethonium is the only example in clinical use. This agonist opens the receptor-operated cation channels on the nicotinic receptor, causing prolonged depolarisation of the membrane around the neuromuscular junction. This stimulates a contraction of the skeletal muscle. However voltage-sensitive sodium channels in other parts of the membrane are rapidly inactivated and action potentials are no longer conducted away from the neuromuscular junction. The muscle becomes unresponsive to the persistent depolarisation at the neuromuscular junction and subsequently relaxes.

Nondepolarising neuromuscular blocking agents, such as vecuronium, are competitive antagonists of acetylcholine at the neuromuscular nicotinic receptor. (Acetylcholine is the excitatory neurotransmitter at the neuromuscular junction.)

Pharmacokinetics: Suxamethonium produces paralysis in about 30 seconds. This is preceded by visible twitching. These features make it ideal for the rapid induction of neuromuscular paralysis which is required prior to intubation in patients who are at risk of aspiration. The action of suxamethonium is terminated by plasma pseudocholinesterases which degrade the drug over 2–3 minutes.

Nondepolarising agents take around 2 minutes to produce complete paralysis. Their action is usually terminated by hepatic metabolism and renal elimination over 20–60 minutes, whereupon further doses may be given with no additional side-effects. Hence they are particularly suitable for maintaining paralysis throughout an operation.

Side-effects: Neuromuscular blocking agents produce complete paralysis of respiratory muscles and are only used by those skilled in artificial ventilation (i.e. anaesthetists). They have no anaesthetic, analgesic or sedative properties. Hence patients must be anaesthetised while neuromuscular paralysis is maintained. Vecuronium has few other side-effects.

Suxamethonium produces muscular pains. It may cause serious hyperkalaemia in patients with burns, renal failure or paraplegia. Repeated injections produce bradycardias by activation of the parasympathetic nervous system. Atropine can prevent this.

Scoline apnoea, phase 2 block and malignant hyperpyrexia are rare but serious reactions to suxamethonium. (See specialised textbooks for further details.)

Reversal of nondepolarising neuromuscular blocking agents

The action of nondepolarising neuromuscular blocking agents can be reversed using acetylcholinesterase inhibitors such as neostigmine. These agents prevent the breakdown of acetylcholine. The increased concentrations of the latter can overcome the action of competitive antagonists such as nondepolarising neuromuscular blocking agents. Neural impulses can then initiate muscular contractions. Acetylcholinesterase inhibitors produce bradycardias by potentiating acetylcholine at parasympathetic ganglia. This is prevented by using muscarinic antagonists such as atropine.

Other nondepolarising blocking agents

Drug	Comment
Atracurium	Degraded in the plasma spontaneously; 20-minute duration. Particularly useful in renal impairment. Causes histamine release
Tubocurarine	Rarely used prototype agent of 45-minute duration. Causes hypotension, histamine release and residual paralysis

Indications for tracheal intubation and neuromuscular paralysis

1. Protection of the respiratory tract from gastric contents. This may arise when the stomach is likely to be full, e.g. urgent operations, any gastrointestinal pathology (including appendicitis), late pregancy, after opioid administration, those in pain.

2. Difficulty maintaining airway using a mask, e.g. patient in prone position, head and neck operations;

3. During mechanical ventilation, especially intrathoracic, abdominal or prolonged operations, or severely ill patients receiving intensive care;

4. Protection of the respiratory tract from blood, e.g. dental and oral procedures.

REVISION AID
Neuromuscular blocking agents

- Neuromuscular blocking agents are used to produce paralysis of voluntary muscles in anaesthetised patients. This prevents reflex movements in response to surgical procedures, including endotracheal intubation, without the need for high concentrations of general anaesthetics

- Neuromuscular blocking agents produce complete paralysis of respiratory muscles and are only used by those skilled in artificial ventilation (i.e. anaesthetists)

- They have no anaesthetic, analgesic or sedative properties and patients must be anaesthetised while neuromuscular paralysis is maintained

- Suxamethonium is a depolarising neuromuscular blocking agent; it acts as an agonist at nicotinic receptors on the neuromuscular junction. Muscular paralysis occurs because voltage-sensitive sodium channels inactivate and fail to conduct action potentials away from the persistently depolarised neuromuscular junctions

- Suxamethonium acts in 30 seconds and is inactivated by plasma pseudocholinesterases after a few minutes. It is ideal for the rapid neuromuscular paralysis required in emergency anaesthesia

- Vecuronium is a nondepolarising neuromuscular blocking agent; it acts as a competitive antagonist of acetylcholine at nicotinic receptors

- Vecuronium acts in 2 minutes and is inactivated over 20 minutes by renal elimination. It is ideal for maintaining paralysis throughout an operation

- The action of nondepolarising neuromuscular blocking agents can be reversed using anticholinesterase inhibitors like neostigmine

32 Local anaesthetic agents: lignocaine

Local anaesthetics, such as lignocaine (also called lidocaine or Xylocaine), are used to provide regional anaesthesia for surgery or pain relief and as antiarrhythmic agents.

Mechanism of action: Local anaesthetics prevent action potential initiation and conductance. They plug the ion channel and prevent conductance through voltage-sensitive sodium channels. They also delay recovery of these channels from their inactivated state and prolong the absolute refractory period (see Fig. 32.1).

Local anaesthetics have basic molecules which access the sodium channel pore from the cytosolic side and must cross the cell membrane to enter the cytosol. The uncharged form of local anaesthetic molecules can cross membranes better. Hence their activity is enhanced at alkaline pH when they are principally in an uncharged state. However it is the charged (cationic) form which actually blocks the sodium channel.

The action of local anaesthetics is use-dependent (the depth of block increases with the frequency of action potentials), partly because they gain access to the channel more readily when it is open, and also because they preferentially bind the channel's inactive state which spontaneously follows its opening.

Local anaesthetics have a greater action on the smaller diameter nerve fibres which carry pain and temperature sensations and regulate blood vessel tone. However, in practice, blockade of most types of sensory and motor neurones occurs.

Pharmacokinetics: Small volumes of local anaesthetics are injected subcutaneously or around nerves. Consequently their local anaesthetic action is usually terminated after 1–2 hours as they are washed into the systemic circulation. Most modern local anaesthetics, such as lignocaine, are amides which are then degraded by liver enzymes, although some short-acting local anaesthetics are esters which are degraded by plasma cholinesterase.

Side-effects: Accidental injection of a bolus of local anaesthetic into the systemic circulation can produce acute toxic effects. These arise from excitation of the central nervous system and depression of the myocardium, causing perioral paraesthesia (tingling around the mouth), agitation, nausea, coma and fits. Fatal cardiac arrhythmias or respiratory arrest may occur if a large volume has been injected.

Hypotension is produced by local anaesthetics, especially when they are used in epidural or spinal techniques (see table 'Local anaesthetic (regional) techniques'), because they block the autonomic control of blood vessel tone. This causes vasodilation in the anaesthetised area. They also reduce cardiac contractility directly by inhibiting sodium entry into cardiac muscle (which will inhibit the sodium–calcium symport and reduce intracellular calcium stores).

Local anaesthetics are rapidly absorbed into the systemic circulation from inflamed and infected tissue and should not be injected into these sites.

Hypersensitivity (allergy) to local anaesthetics occasionally develops, leading to irritation and rashes around the site of injection.

Prolonged anaesthesia may be produced by local anaesthetics. Hence patients should be warned to protect the affected area from trauma or high temperatures for several hours.

Local anaesthetics are often mixed with adrenaline. This prolongs their action by producing local vasoconstriction and preventing washout. However adrenaline can cause arrhythmias and severe hypertension. Hence adrenaline mixtures are avoided in patients with heart disease and for infiltration around fingers, toes and the penis (vasoconstriction of these areas may lead to infarction of the distal tissues).

Other local anaesthetic agents

Drug	Comment
Bupivacaine (Marcaine)	Prolonged action (~8 hours). Widely used for epidurals and postoperative analgesia
Prilocaine	Least toxic agent. Used for Bier's blocks
Cocaine	Causes vasoconstriction. Used to reduce bleeding in nasal operations. Abused by addicts
Procaine	Ester local anaesthetic. Brief action. Rarely used

Local anaesthetic (regional) techniques

Technique	Site of injection	Comment
Local infiltration	Subcutaneous	For surgical incisions
Peripheral nerve block	Around specific nerves	For dental and limb surgery
Bier's block	Veins of a limb isolated from circulation by a pneumatic cuff	Danger of large bolus entering circulation if cuff fails
Spinal anaesthesia	CSF of subarachnoid space	Pelvic and obstetric operations. Causes vasodilation of legs and hypotension
Epidural anaesthesia	Extradural space blocking spinal nerve roots	As spinal. Catheter may be left in place to allow top-up doses

Physiology of sodium channels

Voltage-sensitive sodium channels can exist in three states.

1. Resting; channel can open in response to depolarisation. Depolarisation leads to:

2. open; channel conducts ions. This stage only last 5–10 ms and leads to:

3. inactivated; channel cannot open in response to depolarisation.

The inactivated state will gradually convert to the resting state after the cell has repolarised. The *absolute refractory period* is produced by the existence of this inactivated state. Local anaesthetics plug the open state and delay recovery of the inactivated state to the resting state.

REVISION AID
Local anaesthetic agents

- Local anaesthetics prevent voltage-gated sodium channels opening and stop action potential conduction along nerves

- Their action is use-dependent, it is enhanced at basic pH, and is greater on small diameter fibres

- The action of modern amide local anaesthetics, such as lignocaine, is terminated by tissue washout followed by liver metabolism

- Toxic effects result from accidental release of local anaesthetics into the circulation. These include CNS excitation (including fits), myocardial depression and arrhythmias

- Hypotension occurs when local anaesthetics are used in epidural or spinal techniques because they block the autonomic control of blood pressure

33 Antiepileptic agents: carbamazepine

Epilepsy is characterised by repeated seizures, i.e., transient disturbances of cerebral function due to abnormal electrical discharges. Epilepsy affects 1/200 of the population, and is treated with anticonvulsant drugs such as carbamazepine.

Classification and clinical features:
(See table 'Classification of epilepsy'.)
In primary generalised seizures there is abnormal electrical activity which spreads widely through the brain and is associated with a loss of consciousness. There is no demonstrable focus.

Partial (or focal) seizures are characterised by abnormal electrical activity from a limited region of the brain producing features characteristic of this focus. Consciousness is not lost unless the seizure becomes generalised.

Aetiology: Seizures arise owing to the abnormal repetitive discharge of cerebral neurons. No cause is found in 70% of cases (*primary epilepsy*).

Epilepsy may arise from an imbalance between excitatory and inhibitory neurotransmitters. This causes waves of excitation to spread from the focus to other cortical neurons, producing a seizure. The imbalance may be caused by a defect in brain development.

Many factors can cause secondary epilepsy, including: pathology affecting the brain, (e.g. tumours, or scarring following trauma or anoxia during childbirth); metabolic disorders (such as hypoglycaemia); head injury; intoxication with drugs including local anaesthetics and antidepressants, or sudden withdrawal of antiepileptics or alcohol.

Antiepileptic agents: Carbamazepine is the most widely used antiepileptic drug. The ideal management of recurrent seizures involves the use of a single drug at the lowest effective dose. Unfortunately drug treatment is often lifelong.

Mechanism of action: This is uncertain, although antiepileptic drugs probably block conduction of action potentials away from the epileptic focus. Theories include the following.

1. Inhibition of voltage-dependent sodium channels (e.g. carbamazepine). This prevents depolarisation particularly of the more active neurons around the epileptic focus (use-dependent block). Sodium channel block may also selectively inhibit excitatory amino acid release.

2. Enhancement of the effects of the inhibitory neurotransmitter GABA, either by inhibiting its metabolism or potentiating the chloride flux through the $GABA_A$-receptor chloride channel (e.g. with diazepam).

Pharmacokinetics: Antiepileptic drugs generally have a prolonged action and need to be taken only once or twice a day. However, they are slow to reach a stable plasma concentration. The latter can be measured directly to identify toxicity and poor compliance.

Most antiepileptic drugs strongly induce hepatic enzymes. This reduces the effectiveness of some drugs (e.g. other antiepileptics, oral contraceptives and warfarin).

Side-effects: Most anticonvulsants are sedating and teratogenic. Rashes and blood dyscrasias are common. Acute overdose causes disturbed balance, speech and vision (CNS), and nausea, anorexia and vomiting (GIT). Withdrawal can precipitate seizures.

Vigabatrin: This is a new antiepileptic drug, presently used in combination with other agents for refractory epilepsy. It is an irreversible inhibitor of GABA transaminase and prevents the metabolism of GABA. It is a good example of rational drug design.

Classification of epilepsy

Seizure type	Notes
Generalised	
Tonic–clonic ('grand mal')	Loss of consciousness with stiffness (tonic phase), then rhythmic jerking (clonic phase). Duration ~1–5 minutes
Absence seizures ('petit mal')	Affects children who appear distracted for a few seconds. Treated with ethosuximide and sodium valproate
Partial ('focal') seizures (secondary to local electrical discharge in the brain)	No loss of consciousness. Features depend on location of focus, e.g. motor cortex (jacksonian seizures)

Individual antiepileptic agents

Antiepileptic drug	Mechanism	Notes
Carbamazepine	Blocks sodium channels	Very popular. Least teratogenic
Phenytoin	Blocks sodium channels	Zero-order kinetics. Causes sedation, hirsutism, folate deficiency
Sodium valproate	Uncertain; may enhance GABA or block sodium channels	*Inhibits* hepatic enzymes. Causes hair loss, liver damage (rare)
Ethosuximide	Uncertain; may block calcium channels	Used in absence seizures
Diazepam	Benzodiazepine; enhances GABA	Used i.v. for prolonged seizures (*status epilepticus*)
Vigabatrin	Inhibits GABA metabolism	Used in combinations for refractory epilepsy

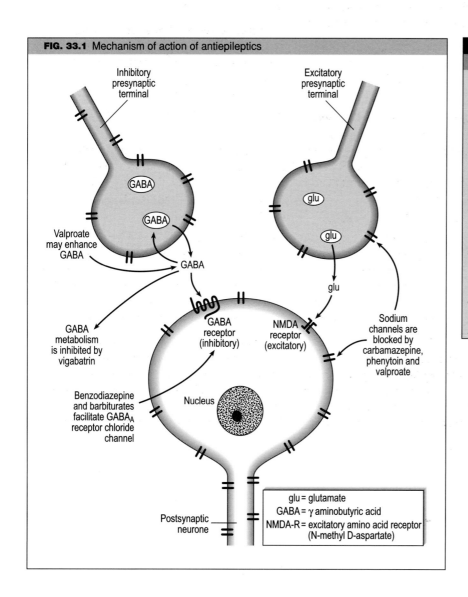

FIG. 33.1 Mechanism of action of antiepileptics

glu = glutamate
GABA = γ aminobutyric acid
NMDA-R = excitatory amino acid receptor (N-methyl D-aspartate)

REVISION AID

Antiepileptic agents

- Epileptic seizures are caused by the abnormal electrical discharge of cortical neurons

- Antiepileptic drugs inhibit the spread of excitation around the epileptic focus. The drugs block sodium channels or enhance the inhibitory neurotransmitter, GABA

- Plasma concentrations of antiepileptics can be measured to identify poor compliance and toxicity

- Side-effects include sedation, teratogenesis, induction of hepatic enzymes and withdrawal seizures. Acute overdose causes CNS and GIT toxicity

34 Drugs used in parkinsonism: L-dopa

Parkinson's disease is a movement disorder caused by a progressive degeneration of the dopaminergic neurons in the substantia nigra. Its prevalence increases with age, affecting 1/200 of people over 70. (Parkinsonism is a syndrome with similar symptoms to Parkinson's disease but with multiple causes.)

Clinical features: Parkinson's disease is characterised by resting tremor, rigidity and bradykinesia (poverty of movement). Difficulty is experienced initiating and terminating voluntary movements. The disease progresses without remission for many years, ultimately causing virtual immobility.

Aetiology: Selective degeneration of neurons in the substantia nigra produces an imbalance of activity between the inhibitory effects of dopamine and the excitatory effects of acetylcholine on neurons within the striatum. The dopaminergic neurons have their cell bodies in the pars compacta of the substantia nigra. Loss of dopaminergic neurons produces an increase in turnover of dopamine in surviving neurons and an increase in dopamine receptors on the postsynaptic

neurons. Multiple subtypes of dopamine receptor are involved. Acetylcholine acts via muscarinic receptors in the striatal nuclei of the basal ganglia. These nuclei are part of the extrapyramidal system.

The reason for the degeneration of dopaminergic neurons in the substantia nigra is not known. An environmental cause, such as a toxin, is suspected, particularly as there is no evidence for a genetic defect. Parkinsonism can result from antipsychotic drugs (which are dopamine antagonists), head injuries, encephalitis and the synthetic neurotoxin MPTP.

Drugs used in parkinsonism: L-dopa

Mechanism of action: Antiparkinsonism drugs act by two main mechanisms:

1. replacing or mimicking the action of dopamine, (e.g. L-dopa); or,
2. using antimuscarinic drugs, antagonising the excitatory action of acetylcholine.

L-dopa is the neutral amino acid precursor of dopamine. L-dopa replenishes dopamine in the striatum.

Pharmacokinetics: L-dopa is rapidly metabolised to dopamine by dopa decarboxylase in the periphery. Hence L-dopa is administered in combination with a peripheral dopa decarboxylase inhibitor such as carbidopa (which remains in the periphery as it is unable to cross the blood–brain barrier). This reduces the required oral dose of L-dopa (as it is being broken down only in the brain), and avoids adverse peripheral effects such as nausea and postural hypotension.

Side-effects: *a. Short-term*: The acute effects of L-dopa are nausea, vomiting and CNS effects such as confusion, hallucinations and dyskinesias (involuntary movements). *b. Long-term*. As Parkinsonism progresses, drugs become less effective. After a number of years of L-dopa treatment episodes of severe immobility and stiffness develop which alternate with dyskinesias (the *on–off effect*). This syndrome can be alleviated by increasing the frequency of drug administration or using additional drugs (see the table 'Other drugs used in parkinsonism').

FIG. 34.1 Control of voluntary movement: the extrapyramidal tract

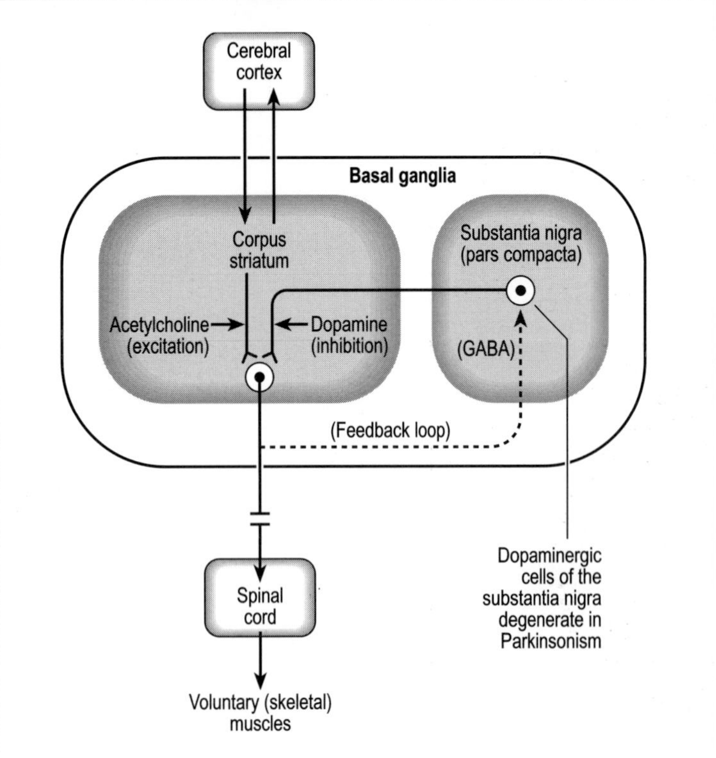

Cerebral cortex

Basal ganglia

Corpus striatum

Substantia nigra (pars compacta)

Acetylcholine (excitation) → ← Dopamine (inhibition)

(GABA)

(Feedback loop)

Spinal cord

Dopaminergic cells of the substantia nigra degenerate in Parkinsonism

Voluntary (skeletal) muscles

Other drugs used in parkinsonism

Drug	Mechanism	Notes
Carbidopa, benserazide	Peripheral dopa decarboxylase inhibitors	Allow reduced L-dopa dose and reduce peripheral side-effects
Selegiline (Deprenyl)	MAO_B inhibitor*	Selectively inhibits dopamine metabolism
Amantadine	Promotes dopamine release	Transient action. GI and CNS side-effects
Benzhexol, procyclidine	Muscarinic antagonists	Used for drug-induced movement disorders
Bromocriptine	Dopamine D_2 agonist	Side-effects similar to those of L-dopa

* Dopamine is selectively metabolised by monoamine oxidase type B (MAO_B)

FIG. 34.2 Mechanism of action of antiparkinsonism drugs: a stylised view of a synapse in the corpus striatum

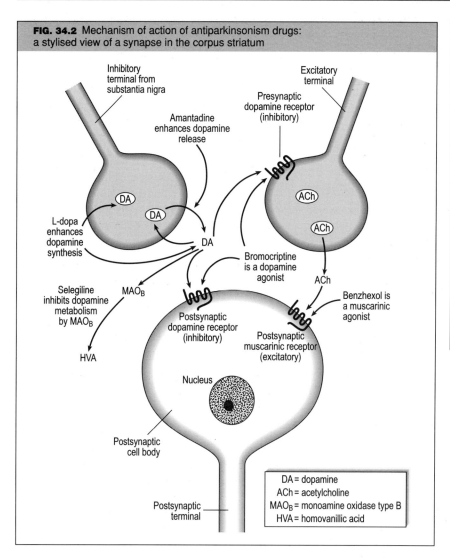

DA = dopamine
ACh = acetylcholine
MAO_B = monoamine oxidase type B
HVA = homovanillic acid

FIG. 34.3 The nigrostriatal dopaminergic pathway

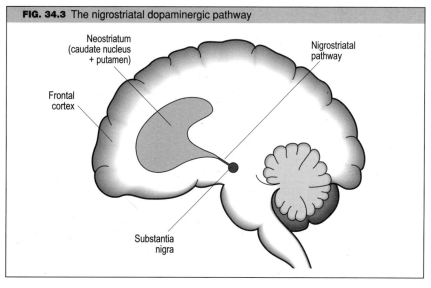

35 Drugs used in migraine: sumatriptan

Migraine is characterised by recurrent headaches associated with visual and gastroenteric disturbances. It is very common, affecting 1/10 of the population.

Clinical features: Symptoms persist for several hours and include headaches of variable severity, either preceded or in conjunction, with episodes including:

1. neurological disturbances such as visual disturbances and photophobia;
2. gastrointestinal disturbances, e.g. nausea and vomiting.

Migraine is disruptive but rarely produces permanent disability.

Aetiology: Migraine has a genetic predisposition. Attacks may be precipitated by factors such as diet, psychological stress and hormonal rhythms. However, the pathophysiology of migraine is unknown.

Many antimigraine drugs interfere with 5-hydroxytryptamine (5-HT) function. Furthermore, agents which release 5-HT can produce migrainous symptoms. An increased blood and urinary release of 5-HT metabolites has been demonstrated during migraine attacks.

One theory suggests that migraine attacks are caused by an excess of 5-HT. This triggers vascular changes such as vasodilation affecting the external cranium, causing headache, and vasoconstriction of intracranial arteries producing cortical ischaemia and neurological features.

Alternatively, spontaneous depression of cortical neurons or the release of neuropeptides may produce secondary neurotransmitter changes, vascular effects and the features of migraine.

Acute treatment: Different drugs are used in the prevention and acute treatment of migraine. Acute treatment may involve the use of simple analgesics like paracetamol. More severe attacks can be treated with specific agents such as sumatriptan.

Mechanism of action: Sumatriptan is a 5-HT_{1D}-receptor agonist which causes vasoconstriction of cranial blood vessels. It is an agonist of 5-HT_{1D}-receptors which are specifically located on cranial vessels. It is not used prophylactically.

Pharmacokinetics: Nausea and vomiting are a common feature of migraine. Hence antimigraine therapy is often given with antiemetics (e.g. metoclopramide).

Side-effects: Sumatriptan is an expensive new agent, of which there is limited clinical experience. However, it is safer than older alternatives. Sumatriptan can produce vascular spasm and must not be used in pregnancy, in patients with cardiovascular disease or for the hemiplegic forms of migraine.

Prophylaxis for migraine: Prophylactic drugs are used if two or more attacks occur each month. Agents such as pizotifen (a 5-HT and H_1-receptor antagonist), propranolol (5-HT_{1D} and β-adrenoreceptor antagonist) and tricyclic antidepressants can be used.

Other antimigraine drugs

Drug	Mechanism	Notes
Acute treatment		
Ergotamine	$5HT_{1D}$, α_1 agonist and directly acting vasoconstrictor	Causes nausea, vomiting, cramps. Tolerance develops. Never use in pregnancy, CVS disease, prophylactically
Prophylaxis		
Pizotifen	$5HT$, H_1 and muscarinic antagonist	Weight gain, antimuscarinic effects
Propranolol	$5HT_{1D}$ and β-antagonist	See Ch. 17, Beta-blockers
Tricyclic antidepressants (e.g. **amitriptyline**)	Inhibit reuptake of neurotransmitters	Antimuscarinic effects
Methysergide	$5HT_2$-antagonist	Specialist use only

REVISION AID

Antimigraine drugs

- Migraines may be due to release of 5-HT and subsequent cerebrovascular changes

- Most antimigraine drugs interfere with 5-HT function

- Acute attacks may be treated with simple analgesics, antiemetics and, in more severe cases, with a vasoconstrictor such as sumatriptan (a 5-HT-receptor agonist)

- Different drugs are used in migraine prophylaxis, such as pizotifen (a 5-HT-receptor antagonist), β-blockers and tricyclic antidepressants

36 Bronchodilators and asthma: salbutamol

Asthma is an inflammatory disease characterised by recurrent reversible obstruction of the airways. It affects 5% of the population and causes wheezing, breathlessness and coughing, particularly in children. Obstruction occurs due to constriction of the bronchioles (bronchospasm) and plugging by excessive secretions. Although asthma is an inflammatory disorder, no allergen is usually identified. Bronchospasm is also a feature of severe allergic, i.e. anaphylactic, reactions and chronic bronchitis. Asthma is treated with bronchodilator drugs. These are often administered using pressurised aerosol inhalers to minimise systemic side-effects.

β_2-Agonists: salbutamol (Ventolin)

Mechanism of action: Salbutamol is an agonist of β_2-adrenoceptors which cause bronchial smooth muscle relaxation and bronchodilation. (There is no sympathetic nerve supply to bronchial smooth muscle. All physiological catecholamine effects are produced by circulating catecholamines.) β_2-Agonists also inhibit mediator release from mast cells.

Pharmacokinetics: Salbutamol can be taken from an inhaler at regular intervals and/or whenever the patient feels breathless. Other drugs are added if a β_2-agonist is required more often than once a day. Salbutamol nebulisers allow concurrent oxygen administration and ensure the drug is being inhaled. Very severe attacks may require salbutamol infusions.

Side-effects: These arise due to systemic β_1- and β_2-adrenoreceptor effects (β_2-agonists are only partially selective). This leads to headache, tremor, tachycardia, palpitations and, at high doses, hypokalaemia.

Sodium cromoglycate

Mechanism of action: Cromoglycate inhalers are used prophylactically, particularly in children because, unlike corticosteroids, cromoglycate does not affect growth. The mechanism of action of cromoglycate is unknown. It may suppress the action of spasmogens from neural or inflammatory cells. Mast cell stabilisation is not important therapeutically.

Side-effects: A cough may result from the inhalation of the dry powder.

Glucocorticoids: beclomethasone
(See also Ch. 41, Glucocorticoids.)

Mechanism of action: Corticosteroids are powerful antiinflammatory drugs. They can be used prophylactically, via inhalers, or systemically in acute attacks.

Side-effects: Inhaled corticosteroids are relatively safe although they may cause oral candidiasis. However, prolonged systemic (i.e. oral) treatment is avoided in all but the most severe cases, as systemic corticosteroids produce multiple severe side-effects.

Other bronchodilator drugs

These include the following.

1. Muscarinic antagonists, such as ipratropium bromide, are particularly useful in chronic bronchitis as they cause bronchodilation and reduce bronchial secretions.

2. Methylxanthines, such as theophylline, prevent breakdown of cAMP and cGMP and act as adenosine receptor antagonists. They are used systemically in severe asthma attacks or in unresponsive cases. Drug interactions and side-effects are common, e.g. gastrointestinal disturbances. Intravenous methylxanthines (aminophylline) may cause convulsions and cardiac arrhythmias.

Asthma attack

With most patients an asthma attack occurs in two distinct phases.

The first phase consists of spasm of the bronchial smooth muscle. Cells such as eosinophils, macrophages and mast cells are all involved in initiating this response via release of spasmogens. These spasmogens include various leukotrienes and histamine. Some of the mediators released also attract leucocytes into the area.

The second phase is an inflammatory reaction. Where infiltration of inflammatory cells (leucocytes) occurs, including infiltration by T cells and eosinophils. T cells secrete cytokines (important mediators of inflammatory and immune responses), whilst the eosinophils secrete various proteins which can damage the epithelial layer.

Anti-asthma drugs

Drugs used to treat asthma can be classified into two broad groups, anti-inflammatory agents and bronchodilators. Anti-inflammatory drugs act in both phases to combat the inflammatory agents. Bronchodilators act in primarily the first phase to counteract the bronchospasm.

Bronchodilators include: β_2-adrenoceptor agonists, methylxanthines and anti-muscarinics.

Anti-inflammatory agents include: glucocorticoids, sodium cromoglycate, H_1 antagonists (anti-histamines)

REVISION AID
Bronchodilators and asthma

- Asthma is an inflammatory disease characterised by reversible obstruction of the airways due to bronchoconstriction and mucous plugging

- Bronchodilator drugs are often administered by inhalers although more severe attacks require use of nebulisers or systemic routes. Examples include:

  1. β_2-adrenoceptor agonists, e.g. salbutamol
  2. Sodium cromoglycate (prophylaxis only)
  3. Corticosteroids, e.g. beclomethasone
  4. Muscarinic antagonists
  5. Methylxanthines

- β_2-adrenoceptor agonists produce side-effects such as headache, tremor, palpitations and, at high doses, hypokalaemia

- If β_2-adrenoceptor agonists are required more often than once a day, then other agents should be added such as inhaled cromoglycate or corticosteroids

37 Drugs used in peptic ulcer disease: cimetidine

A peptic ulcer is a breach in the lining (mucosa) of the stomach or the first part of the duodenum. The lower oesophagus may be involved if there is an incompetent gastrooesophageal sphincter. The aetiology of peptic ulcer disease is uncertain although excessive gastric acid secretion and infection with *Helicobacter pylori* are probably important factors. Peptic ulcers may be aggravated by smoking, alcohol abuse or NSAIDs. The symptoms produced by these conditions include epigastric pain, heartburn and indigestion. Many antiulcer drugs reduce gastric acid secretion. Eradication of *Helicobacter pylori* using antibiotics and bismuth chelates prevents recurrence of peptic ulcers.

H$_2$-receptor antagonists: cimetidine

Mechanism of action: These drugs heal peptic ulcers by reducing gastric acid secretion. They are selective antagonists of histamine H$_2$-receptors on the acid-secreting parietal cells of the stomach. They have little effect on H$_1$-receptors.

Pharmacokinetics: H$_2$-receptor antagonists heal ulcers in 4–8 weeks. They are usually administered orally at night. There is a high relapse rate so treatment may be required indefinitely. Cimetidine inhibits hepatic drug metabolism and should be avoided in combination with warfarin, some antiepileptics or bronchodilators.

Side-effects: These are uncommon but may include dizziness, fatigue, headache, rashes and (very rarely) renal and hepatic impairment. If given intravenously, they should be infused slowly in dilute solutions to avoid cardiac arrhythmias. Cimetidine can produce gynaecomastia (enlargement of the male breast).

Proton-pump inhibitors: omeprazole

Mechanism of action: Omeprazole inhibits gastric acid secretion by irreversibly blocking the hydrogen–potassium active transporter on parietal cells.

Pharmocokinetics: Omeprazole is activated at low pH. Consequently its actions are specific to the very acidic conditions around gastric parietal cells.

Side-effects: Diarrhoea, rashes and headache may occur.

Antacids: aluminium hydroxide and magnesium hydroxide

Mechanism of action: Antacids are basic compounds which chemically neutralise gastric acid. They relieve the symptoms of peptic ulcer disease.

Pharmacokinetics: They are taken as tablets or suspensions either acutely or just before symptoms are expected (usually between meals and at bedtime). Patients with recurrent symptoms may require administration at regular, even hourly, intervals.

They impair the absorption of other drugs and should not be taken concurrently.

Side-effects: See table 'Side-effects of antacids'.

Other antiulcer drugs: See table 'Drugs used in peptic ulcer disease'.

Inflammatory bowel disease: ulcerative colitis and Crohn's disease

Ulcerative colitis is an inflammatory condition of unknown aetiology. It produces an inflammation of the large bowel mucosa, causing diarrhoea which contains blood and mucus.

Crohn's disease can affect any part of the gastrointestinal tract but has a predilection for the small bowel and colon. In Crohn's disease the whole thickness of the bowel wall is inflamed. This causes diarrhoea, abdominal pain and weight loss. Complications include strictures, fistulae, abscesses and adhesions.

Corticosteroids are important in the treatment of inflammatory bowel disease. They can be administered topically to the rectum (as enemas) or systemically.

For more extensive disease, salicylic acid combinations (such as sulphasalazine) are used to maintain remissions. These agents modify the immune response (see Ch. 42, Drugs used in rheumatoid arthritis). Salicylates can produce diarrhoea, allergies and renal damage.

See also the table 'Salicylates used in inflammatory bowel disease'.

Drugs used in peptic ulcer disease

Drug	Mechanism	Side-effects	Comments
Cimetidine	H_2-receptor antagonist	Uncommon – gynaecomastia	Inhibits hepatic drug metabolism
Ranitidine	H_2-receptor antagonist	Uncommon	
Omeprazole	Proton pump inhibitor	Diarrhoea and headaches	Inhibits parietal cell H^+/K^+ active transporter
Misoprostol	Prostaglandin E analogue	Diarrhoea	Prevents NSAID-induced ulcers
Pirenzepine	Selective muscarinic M_1-antagonist	Peripheral antimuscarinic effects	Cannot cross blood–brain barrier
Sucralfate (aluminium and sulphated sucrose complex)	Forms protective barrier on gastric mucosa. (Minimal antacid action)	GI disturbances	Nasogastric tube administration on Intensive Care (prevents stress ulcers)
Bismuth chelates	Eradicate *H. pylori* and promotes prostaglandin E and bicarbonate release	Darkens tongue and blackens faeces	Can be used with antibiotics to eradicate *H. pylori*

Side-effects of antacids

Constituent	Side-effect
Aluminium	Constipation
Magnesium	Diarrhoea
Bicarbonates	Belching (from carbon dioxide release)
Sodium	Water retention, aggravates heart failure

Salicylates used in inflammatory bowel disease

Drug	Constituents
Sulphasalazine	5-aminosalicylic acid + sulphapyridine
Mesalazine	5-aminosalicylic acid
Olsalazine	5-aminosalicylic acid dimer

FIG. 37.1 Drugs used in the treatment of peptic ulcer disease

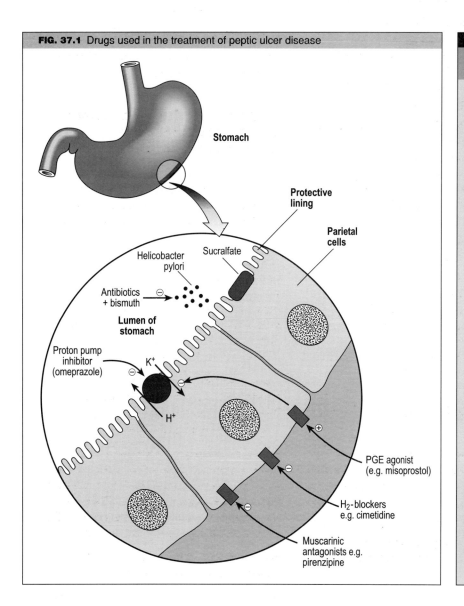

Drugs used in peptic ulcer disease

- A peptic ulcer is an erosion of the lining (mucosa) of the stomach or duodenum which arises from excess gastric acid secretion

- Antagonists of histamine H_2-receptors reduce gastric acid secretion (e.g. cimetidine). They have few side-effects although recurrences occur on withdrawal

- Other agents which reduce gastric acid secretion in peptic ulcer disease include: the proton pump inhibitor, omeprazole; prostaglandin E agonists, and muscarinic M_1-receptor antagonists. Other drugs produce a protective barrier over the gastric mucosa or eradicate *Helicobacter pylori*

- Antacids, e.g. aluminium hydroxide and magnesium hydroxide, relieve the symptoms of peptic ulcer disease. They neutralise gastric acid. They may cause constipation or diarrhoea

- Inflammatory bowel disease (ulcerative colitis and Crohn's disease) causes chronic diarrhoea and abdominal pain. Corticosteroids are used during exacerbations, and salicylate combinations for maintenance

38. Laxatives and antidiarrhoeals: lactulose and codeine

Laxatives

Laxatives are used to treat constipation, i.e. the passage of hard stools and less frequently than usual for an individual. However any underlying cause must be identified and treated. Attention to diet, fluid consumption and reassurance mean laxatives can usually be avoided, except in the prevention of drug-induced constipation or where straining exacerbates other conditions, e.g. haemorrhoids and angina.

Pharmacokinetics: Laxatives are usually taken orally although some stimulant laxatives are available as suppositories or enemas.

Side-effects: Many laxatives stimulate intestinal peristalsis. This may produce abdominal cramps and may even cause bowel perforation in patients with intestinal obstruction. Excessive use of laxatives may cause hypokalaemia and further impair the functions of the colon.

Osmotic laxatives, e.g. lactulose: These agents cannot be digested or absorbed and therefore retain fluid in the bowel by osmosis. This increases faecal bulk and softens and lubricates stools. Lactulose is a synthetic disaccharide.

Bulk-forming laxatives, e.g. bran: Bran cannot be digested and therefore increases faecal bulk. This softens hard stools and gradually stimulates peristalsis. These preparations swell in contact with liquids and may produce intestinal obstruction unless adequate fluids are consumed. Some bulk-forming laxatives must be reconsituted with water.

Liquid paraffin: This is a faecal softener. It causes anal seepage and irritation.

Stimulant laxatives: These agents are administered orally or rectally and irritate the intestinal mucosa, thereby stimulating fluid secretion and peristalsis. They are very powerful and are seldom required. They are used in terminal care and to evacuate the bowel prior to surgery or diagnostic examinations.

Parasympathomimetics: These produce similar effects to stimulant laxatives. They include muscarinic agonists and acetylcholinesterase inhibitors.

Antidiarrhoeal drugs: codeine phosphate

Diagnosis of any underlying pathology, and fluid and salt replacement are important considerations in treating diarrhoea. Most cases of diarrhoea follow viral infection and resolve quickly. Hence antidiarrhoeal drugs are seldom required other than to relieve abdominal cramps or to provide temporary relief, e.g. to permit an important journey.

Occasionally bacterial diarrhoea may require antibiotic agents. (Paradoxically, diarrhoea is a side-effect of antibiotic use.)

Bulk-forming laxatives: These may help to control diarrhoea, because they increase faecal bulk, particularly in patients with diverticular disease.

Antimotility drugs: These include opioids and antimuscarinics (muscarinic antagonists). Opioids (such as codeine) produce disorganised peristaltic contractions and reduce intestinal motility. Although they increase the activity of intestinal smooth muscle, these contractions no longer transport the luminal contents effectively.

Antispasmodics: These are used to relieve the cramps associated with diarrhoea and other intestinal disease. They relax gastrointestinal smooth muscle either by a direct action or by inhibiting the actions of the parasympathetic nervous system (e.g. antimuscarinics).

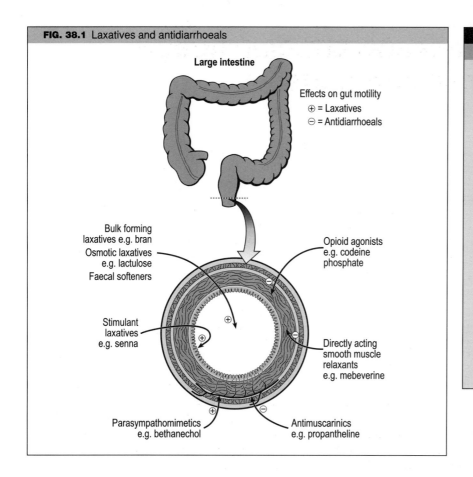

FIG. 38.1 Laxatives and antidiarrhoeals

Large intestine

Effects on gut motility
⊕ = Laxatives
⊖ = Antidiarrhoeals

Bulk forming
laxatives e.g. bran
Osmotic laxatives
e.g. lactulose
Faecal softeners

Opioid agonists
e.g. codeine
phosphate

Stimulant
laxatives
e.g. senna

Directly acting
smooth muscle
relaxants
e.g. mebeverine

Parasympathomimetics
e.g. bethanechol

Antimuscarinics
e.g. propantheline

Examples of laxatives

Mechanism of action	Examples
Osmotic laxatives	Lactulose, magnesium salts, rectal sodium and phosphate salts
Bulk-forming laxatives	Bran, methylcellulose (also used in diarrhoea)
Faecal softener	Liquid paraffin
Stimulant laxatives	Senna, glycerol suppositories, sodium picosulphate
Parasympathomimetics	
Muscarinic agonist	Bethanechol
Acetylcholinesterase inhibitor	Neostigmine

Examples of antidiarrhoeals

Mechanism of action	Examples
Antimotility drugs: opioid agonists	Codeine phosphate, loperamide (no CNS penetration)
Antispasmodics	
Antimuscarinic	Propantheline
Directly acting smooth muscle relaxant	Mebeverine

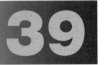

Diabetes mellitus:
insulin and gliclazide

Aetiology and classification: Type 1 diabetes occurs where there is a complete loss of insulin from the pancreatic beta cells. It can only be treated with insulin. Type 2 diabetes is due to variable degrees of insulin deficiency and tissue unresponsiveness (insulin resistance). Type 2 diabetes can be treated with diet, oral hypoglycaemic drugs and/or insulin (see the table 'Features of types 1 and 2 diabetes'). Diabetes disrupts carbohydrate, protein and fat metabolism to produce complications in every organ of the body.

Clinical features: Diabetes is diagnosed by demonstrating a random blood glucose level greater than 11 mmol/L. Presenting symptoms include excessive thirst, urinary frequency, fatigue, infections (especially on the skin or urinary tract) and blurred vision. Type 1 diabetes occurs in younger people and may present suddenly, with life-threatening ketoacidosis (see the table, 'Clinical features of diabetes'). Type 2 diabetes is more common and usually occurs in older people where insulin resistance produces hyperglycaemia. Patients may present with mild weight loss, urinary symptoms or chronic diabetic complications (see table) or diabetes may be detected by incidental screening for urinary glucose.

Insulin

Mechanism of action: Insulin is used to supplement or replace the insulin deficiency

present in diabetes. It is the only treatment for type 1 diabetes. Insulin acts at membrane-bound receptors which exhibit tyrosine kinase activity and activate the MAP–kinase pathway. Insulin therefore regulates gene expression in a manner similar to that of many growth hormones. (See the table 'Actions of insulin' for a summary.)

Pharmacokinetics: Most proprietary insulin formulations are structurally identical to human insulin. They may be short-, intermediate- or long-acting (see the table 'Pharmacokinetics of subcutaneous insulin formations'). For routine maintenance, mixtures of 2/3 intermediate-acting and 1/3 short-acting insulin are injected subcutaneously. Typically, 2/3 of the daily dose is taken before breakfast and 1/3 before the evening meal. Short-acting (or soluble) insulin is given intravenously in diabetic emergencies, such as ketoacidosis, or during labour.

Side-effects: The dose and frequency of insulin injections are adjusted to reduce variations in blood glucose as far as possible. This minimises the acute and chronic complications of diabetes, especially hypoglycaemia (see table 'Clinical features of diabetes'). Immunological resistance to insulin is uncommon. However fat hypertrophy can occur at injection sites.

Oral hypoglycaemics: gliclazide

Mechanism of action: Sulphonylureas, such as gliclazide, stimulate pancreatic insulin release and are therefore only useful in type 2 diabetes. They act on membrane-bound receptors and thereby inhibit ATP-dependent potassium channels, causing cellular depolarisation and increasing insulin secretion.

Pharmacokinetics: Longer acting hypoglycaemics only need to be given once a day. However this predisposes elderly patients to hypoglycaemia, so shorter acting agents, like gliclazide, are preferable.

Side-effects: Weight gain, hypoglycaemia, gastrointestinal disturbances and headaches.

Metformin: This biguanide is an oral hypoglycaemic which is more suitable for obese type 2 diabetics as it may suppress appetite. It increases peripheral uptake of glucose and reduces hepatic output. It may cause gastrointestinal disturbances and, rarely, it may precipitate lactic acidosis (a very serious complication).

REVISION AID

Diabetes mellitus

- Type 1 diabetes is due to deficiency of insulin. It can only be treated with insulin

- Type 2 diabetes is due to variable degrees of insulin deficiency or resistance. It can be treated with diet, oral hypoglycaemic drugs and/or insulin

- Diabetes disrupts carbohydrate, protein and fat metabolism to produce complications in every organ of the body

- Insulin receptors exhibit tyrosine kinase activity and activate the MAP–kinase pathway thereby regulating gene expression

- Insulin is usually injected subcutaneously, twice daily before meals

- The dose, formulation and frequency of administration is adjusted to minimise variations in blood glucose, thereby minimising diabetic complications

- Oral hypoglycaemics are only useful in type 2 diabetes. Their main side-effect is hypoglycaemia

- Sulphonylureas, such as gliclazide, stimulate pancreatic insulin release

Features of types 1 and 2 diabetes

Feature	Type 1	Type 2
Loss of insulin secretion	Total	Partial
Insulin resistance	None	Present
Treatment	Insulin	Diet, oral hypoglycaemics and/or insulin
Age at onset	Young	Middle-age or older
Aetiology	Genetic/autoimmune	Genetic
Precipitants	? Viral infection	Obesity, high carbohydrate diet, thiazide diuretics, β-blockers

Pharmacokinetics of subcutaneous insulin formulations

Formulation	Onset	Maximum effects, hours	Duration, hours
Short-acting (soluble)	30–60 minutes	2–4	~8
Intermediate- and long-acting	1–2 hours	4–8	16–35

Actions of insulin

Insulin receptors: These are located in the membranes of fat, muscle, liver and brain cells. Insulin receptors become internalised after agonist occupation. They exhibit tyrosine kinase activity and activate the MAP–kinase pathway which alters gene expression

Actions: Insulin activates anabolic processes and inhibits catabolism. It promotes cellular uptake of glucose, amino acids and fatty acids

Effects include:

- Liver: stimulates glycogen synthesis; inhibits ketone formation

- Skeletal muscle: stimulates glucose uptake; stimulates glycogen synthesis

- Adipose tissue: stimulates glucose uptake; inhibits lipolysis

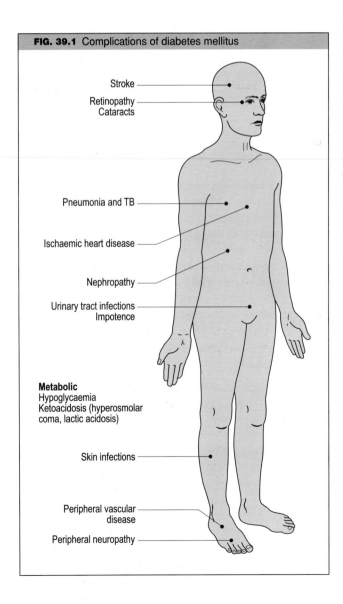

FIG. 39.1 Complications of diabetes mellitus

Stroke
Retinopathy
Cataracts

Pneumonia and TB

Ischaemic heart disease

Nephropathy

Urinary tract infections
Impotence

Metabolic
Hypoglycaemia
Ketoacidosis (hyperosmolar coma, lactic acidosis)

Skin infections

Peripheral vascular disease
Peripheral neuropathy

Clinical features of diabetes

Presenting features: These are as follows.

- Type 1 diabetes: young adults, excessive thirst, urinary frequency, fatigue, infections (especially on the skin or urinary tract) and blurred vision; or ketoacidosis

- Type 2 diabetes: older patients, mild weight loss or urinary symptoms, chronic diabetic complications; asymptomatic but detected by screening for glucose in the urine

Acute complications: These are all emergencies and require biochemical tests to confirm the diagnosis and guide management

- Hypoglycaemia (insulin overdose)
  a. Features of sympathetic overactivity: hunger, agitation, sweating, pallor, palpitations
  b. Features of cerebral glycopenia: dizziness, headaches, confusion or coma

- Ketoacidosis (type 1 diabetes): dehydration, vomiting, rapid breathing with the smell of ketones on breath, confusion or coma

- Rare emergencies include: hyperosmolar coma (type 2 diabetes) and lactic acidosis (complication of biguanide treatment)

Chronic complications: These may be avoided by minimising fluctuations in plasma glucose.

- Cataracts, retinopathy, foot ulcers, ischaemic vascular disease (including heart attacks and peripheral vascular disease), neurological disease (strokes, peripheral and autonomic neuropathies), renal failure

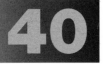

Oral contraceptives: ethinyloestradiol and norethisterone

Oral contraception is the use of orally active sex hormones to prevent pregnancy while allowing intercourse to take place. Around 3 million British women currently use them.

Mechanism of action: Combined oral contraceptive (COC) preparations are the most popular. They contain an oestrogen, usually ethinyloestradiol, with one of six progestogens, e.g. norethisterone. These steroid hormones act on intracellular receptors to regulate gene transcription. Ovulation is prevented by inhibition of pituitary luteinising hormone (LH) and follicle-stimulating hormone (FSH) release (see tables 'Actions of oestrogens' and 'Actions of progestogens').

Pharmacokinetics: Continuous hormone exposure produces irregular bleeding. Hence hormones are administered for 21 days followed by a 7-day break to permit predictable withdrawal bleeding and minimise the overall exposure to hormones. Low dose preparations are preferable as side-effects are reduced.

Side-effects: Oral contraceptives are extremely safe for most women. (Their use confers less risk than having a baby or an abortion.) However they are contraindicated in pregnancy, serious cardiovascular disease and in women with a history of thromboemboli (e.g. pulmonary emboli, deep vein thromboses). COCs should be stopped 4 weeks prior to major surgery.

COCs produce a fourfold increase in incidence of thromboemboli (particularly those COCs containing the newer progestogens). COCs may increase the risk of carcinoma of the breast and cervix. They aggravate inflammatory bowel disease and migraine.

Temporary side-effects include headaches, breast tenderness and irregular bleeding. Breakthrough bleeding may be relieved by using a higher dose of progestogens.

Other side-effects include impaired lactation, fluid retention, weight gain, gallstones, mood changes and adverse effects on serum lipid profiles.

Advantages of COCs compared to other contraceptives: These include a low failure rate, and reduced incidences of ovarian and endometrial cancer, menorrhagia, dysmenorrhoea, iron deficiency anaemia, benign breast disease, pelvic inflammatory disease and ovarian cysts. They may protect against thyroid disease, rheumatoid arthritis, fibroids and osteroporosis.

Interactions of oral contraceptives: Antibiotics may cause diarrhoea and destroy the gut bacteria that recycle metabolised oestrogens. Some drugs, especially antiepileptics, induce hepatic metabolism of steroid hormones. These make oral contraceptives less efficient, and higher dose pills or alternative methods are required. Alternative methods are also needed following diarrhoea, vomiting and emergency contraception.

Procedures for missed pills: Alternative methods should be used for 7 days if a COC is taken more than 12 hours late, or if a progestogen-only pill (POP) is taken more than 3 hours late.

Progestogen-only pills ('minipills'): These provide continous exposure to progestogens. POPs make cervical mucus relatively impermeable to sperm, render the endometrium unsuitable for implantation and alter the motility of the fallopian tubes (which normally directs the egg or conceptus from the ovary to the uterus). They are used to avoid oestrogen administration in smokers aged over 35, and those with hypertension, heart disease, diabetes or migraine.

POPs do not increase the rates of thrombosis. However, they have a higher failure rate and produce irregular bleeding. They must be taken within a 3-hour period on each day as their effects only last for 24 hours. Hence progestogen injections and implants are becoming popular. POPs do not prevent lactation and can be used in nursing mothers.

Emergency contraception (the 'morning-after pill')

This involves the administration of two doses, exactly 12 hours apart, within 72 hours of a single episode of unprotected intercourse. These preparations contain high concentrations of oestrogens and progestogens which prevent implantation of the conceptus. Side-effects are similar to COCs. However nausea and vomiting are more common and alternative contraception must be used for 7 days.

Alternatively an intrauterine device (the coil) may be inserted. This is more reliable than the morning-after pill.

Actions of oestrogens

1. Secondary sexual characteristics: breast and genital development.

2. Menstruation functions:
   a. inhibit FSH release; inhibit LH and gonadotrophin-releasing hormone (GnRH) release at low concentrations; stimulate LH and GnRH release at high concentrations
   b. promote maturation of oocyte
   c. cyclical development of breasts and uterus.

3. Metabolic effects:
   a. increase clotting factors 7, 8, 9 and 10 and inhibit fibrinolysis
   b. increase serum renin, angiotensin, thyroxine and cortisol
   c. reduce peripheral glucose uptake
   d. increase serum cholesterol and triglycerides; reduce serum HDL
   e. promote bone calcification and reduce serum and urine calcium.

4. Oestrogen priming is needed for progesterone receptor synthesis and responses.

Hormone replacement therapy (HRT)

This is intended to replace the deficiency of female sex hormones in postmenopausal women. To minimise side-effects, lower doses of naturally occurring hormones (such as oestradiol) are used. HRT increases the risk of endometrial and, possibly, breast carcinoma. Weight gain and continued menstrual bleeding may be a problem. There is no increased risk of cervix or ovarian cancer, hypertension or thromboemboli. The benefits of HRT usually outweigh these risks.

Benefits of HRT: These include:

1. relief from symptoms of menopause

2. reduction in incidence of osteoporotic fractures by 50% over 5 years

3. reduced risk of heart disease, partly by reducing serum LDL cholesterol.

Actions of progestogens

1. Inhibit FSH release, LH and GnRH release.

2. Cervical mucus becomes thicker, opaque and less abundant.

3. Promote secretory changes in endometrium, glandular development of breasts and reduce uterine excitability.

4. Relax smooth muscle in general.

5. Metabolic effects:
   a. increase body temperature
   b. promote sodium excretion (by opposing aldosterone)
   c. increase respiratory minute volume (reduce arterial CO_2)
   d. promote protein catabolism and nitrogen excretion.

Hormonal control of the female reproductive system

1. The menstrual cycle starts with menstruation.

2. GnRH is released in pulses from the hypothalamus and acts on the pituitary to release FSH and LH, which then act on the ovary.

3. FSH stimulates follicle development. FSH is the main hormone controlling oestrogen secretion. LH stimulates ovulation at midcycle. LH is the main hormone controlling subsequent progesterone secretion from the corpus luteum.

4. Oestogen controls the early, proliferative phase during which the endometrium proliferates and progestogen receptors appear on target tissues. Progestogen controls the later, secretory phase (which follows ovulation), during which the endometrium becomes suitable for implantation and support of the conceptus. Both have negative feedback effects on the hypothalamus and anterior pituitary which prevent further ovulations.

5. If a fertilised ovum is implanted, the corpus luteum continues to secrete progestogens during the pregnancy. If no fertilised ovum implants, the corpus luteum degenerates, progestogen levels fall and the endometrium sloughs away causing menstruation.

Oral contraceptives

- Combined oral contraceptive preparations (COCs) prevent ovulation

- They contain an oestrogen, usually ethinyloestradiol and a progestogen, e.g. norethisterone

- They are administered for 21 days followed by a 7-day break

- COCs increase the risk of thromboemboli. However they improve or prevent many other conditions

- The effectiveness of COCs can be reduced by diarrhoea, vomiting, antibiotics, drugs which induce hepatic enzymes, and emergency oral contraception

- Progesterone-only pills (POPs) prevent sperm passing through the cervix and prevent implantation of the conceptus, by effects on the cervical mucus, the endometrium and the fallopian tubes

- POPs have a higher failure rate than COCs but are more suitable for women with cardiovascular risk factors or those with oestrogen intolerance

41 Glucocorticoids: hydrocortisone

Steroids such as glucocorticoids and reproductive hormones are synthesised from cholesterol. Glucocorticoid hormones such as hydrocortisone (cortisol) are secreted from the zona fasciculata of the adrenal cortex.

Mechanism of action: Glucocorticoids bind intracellular receptors and modulate gene transcription by directly interacting with sites on DNA. Immunosuppression is their main therapeutic use, although the onset of this effect takes 2–4 hours. Glucocorticoids inhibit the proliferation of immune cells and their functions (such as phagocytosis and release of lysosomal enzymes). Mechanisms implicated include the inhibition of synthesis of immune modulators such as prostaglandins, leukotrienes and interleukins. For example, prostaglandin synthesis is reduced, as glucocorticoids inhibit expression of cyclooxygenase and phospholipase A_2.

Glucocorticoids produce atrophy of lymphoid tissues such as lymph nodes, thymus, tonsils and spleen. They reduce scar tissue formation by inhibiting fibroblasts and mucopolysaccharide synthesis. This also delays wound healing. For other physiological actions and therapeutic uses see the tables 'Main actions of glucocorticoids' and 'Conditions where glucocorticoids are used'.

Pharmacokinetics: Prolonged systemic administration of glucocorticoids is avoided because these drugs have many serious side-effects. Hence they may be administered, using inhalers or nebulisers (for asthma), by injection into joints (for rheumatoid arthritis), as skin creams (for eczema) and as rectal foams and enemas (for inflammatory bowel disease).

Adrenal suppression is avoided by administration as a single daily dose in the morning and using intermittent, short courses.

Side-effects: Acute glucocorticoid administration produces few side-effects. Chronic administration produces the following.

1. Suppression of hypothalamic corticotrophin-releasing factor and pituitary ACTH. This leads to adrenal atrophy and an inability to secrete physiological quantities of glucocorticoids. If chronic administration is suddenly stopped there may be an Addisonian crisis (hypotension and cardiovascular collapse due to inadequate glucocorticoid levels). The adrenals can recover if glucocorticoids are gradually withdrawn over several weeks. An increase in maintenance doses is also needed temporarily following stresses, such as surgery, which normally increase glucocorticoid output.

2. Sodium and water retention due to mineralocorticoid actions. This exacerbates heart failure and causes oedema and hypertension.

3. Immune suppression predisposing to infections such as acne and TB.

4. Changes in carbohydrate metabolism causing hyperglycaemia which may precipitate diabetes.

5. Changes in fat metabolism causing central fat deposition with facial roundness, buffalo humps and obesity.

6. Increased tissue and protein metabolism causing growth retardation, proximal muscle wasting, osteoporosis and fractures, skin thinning and fragility (leading to stretch marks and bruising) and impaired wound healing.

7. Other side-effects, including amenorrhoea, peripheral neuropathy, psychoses and depression, peptic ulcers, cataracts and glaucoma.

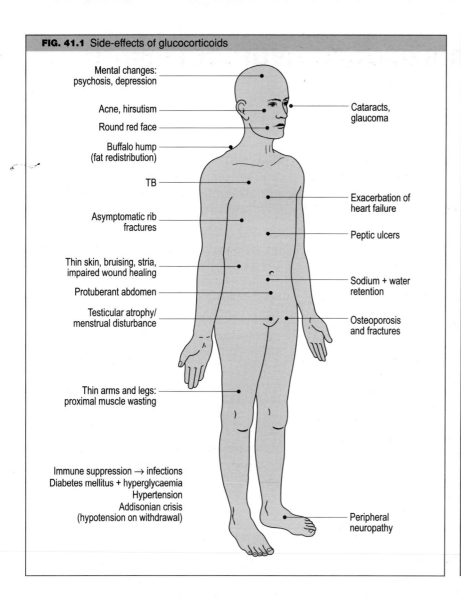

FIG. 41.1 Side-effects of glucocorticoids

Mental changes: psychosis, depression

Acne, hirsutism

Round red face

Buffalo hump (fat redistribution)

TB

Asymptomatic rib fractures

Thin skin, bruising, stria, impaired wound healing

Protuberant abdomen

Testicular atrophy/ menstrual disturbance

Thin arms and legs: proximal muscle wasting

Immune suppression → infections
Diabetes mellitus + hyperglycaemia
Hypertension
Addisonian crisis
(hypotension on withdrawal)

Cataracts, glaucoma

Exacerbation of heart failure

Peptic ulcers

Sodium + water retention

Osteoporosis and fractures

Peripheral neuropathy

Glucocorticoids

- Glucocorticoid hormones such as hydrocortisone (cortisol) are secreted from the adrenal cortex

- Their actions include effects on carbohydrate, fat and protein metabolism. They are used clinically to suppress inflammatory responses including autoimmune responses and scar formation

- They are used locally to treat rheumatoid arthritis, asthma, inflammatory bowel disease and eczema

- Glucocorticoids activate intracellular receptors which bind sites on DNA and induce gene transcription

- They have many side-effects, particularly following chronic, systemic use, and they are administered by local application whenever possible

- Chronic glucocorticoid treatment must be withdrawn gradually

- Temporarily increased doses are needed following surgery or other stresses

- Side-effects include adrenal suppression, susceptibility to infections, salt and water retention (which aggravates heart failure) and osteoporosis

Main actions of glucocorticoids

1. Carbohydrate metabolism: increase blood glucose by stimulating glycogenesis and gluconeogenesis

2. Protein metabolism: increase protein breakdown (catabolism)

3. Fat metabolism: increase lipolysis of peripheral fat depots and deposition on the trunk

4. Suppression of inflammation: inhibition of many immunological functions including acute immune responses and delayed responses (such as scar formation)

5. Endocrine: suppression of pituitary ACTH, LH, FSH, thyroid-stimulating hormone (TSH) and growth hormone (GH) release

6. Mineralocorticoid effects (potassium excretion, salt and water retention)

7. Permissive actions on adrenaline and insulin

8. Reduce calcium absorption and increase secretion

Conditions where glucocorticoids are used

- CVS: rheumatic carditis, myocarditis

- Respiratory system: asthma, pulmonary fibrosis

- Gut: exacerbations of inflammatory bowel disease

- Renal: nephrotic syndrome (autoimmune condition directed against the kidneys)

- CNS: prevention of scarring and cerebral oedema produced by surgery, head injuries and tumours; exacerbations of multiple sclerosis; temporal arteritis

- Musculoskeletal system: rheumatoid arthritis and other collagen–vascular diseases

- Eye: prevention of scarring following surgery and uveitis

- Skin: eczema; severe inflammatory skin conditions including pemphigus

- Endocrine: replacement therapy in Addison's disease

- Immune system: anaphylactic shock (severe allergic reactions); prevention of transplanted organ rejection

- Blood: autoimmune anaemia and thrombocytopenia (platelet deficiency); leukaemia and Hodgkin's disease

Examples of glucocorticoid hormones

Glucocorticoid	Comment
Hydrocortisone	Popular intravenous formulation
Prednisolone	Popular oral formulation
Dexamethasone	Potent oral formulation (lacks mineralocorticoid activity)
Beclomethasone	Inhaled or topical

42 Drugs used in rheumatoid arthritis: sulphasalazine

Rheumatoid arthritis is a chronic systemic disease producing inflammation and progressive destruction of the joints and damage to many other organs. It affects ~2% of the population and is more common in women.

Clinical features: Rheumatoid arthritis typically produces pain and stiffness in the small joints especially the knuckles. Progressive inflammation causes irreversible erosion, deformity and instability of the joints. Tendon sheaths are also damaged, further disrupting the joints. Extra-articular manifestations include effusion of fluid around the lungs and heart, leg ulcers, dryness and inflammation of the eyes, anaemia and immune deficiency. The nervous system may be damaged by entrapment in tendons or dislocation of vertebrae.

Aetiology: The cause of rheumatoid arthritis is unknown. There is a genetic predisposition, and it is associated with the expression of certain human leucocyte antigens (HLA-DR4). There are many immunological disturbances. Chronic inflammatory processes which are directed against the synovium may be initiated by a foreign antibody (such as a virus). Toxic inflammatory mediators are then released which progressively erode the articular cartilage.

Management: Physiotherapy, splints and corrective surgery are all important in the management of rheumatoid arthritis. Drug treatment begins with NSAIDs (such as aspirin) to relieve joint pain. NSAIDs are no longer thought to modify the disease progression (see Ch. 28, Nonsteroidal antiinflammatory drugs). Side-effects are minimised by employing slow-release formulations and antiulcer drugs. Exacerbations or arthritis may be treated using corticosteroid joint injection.

Prolonged oral corticosteroid treatment produces many severe side-effects and is reserved for extreme cases (see Ch. 41, Glucocorticoids).

Specific antirheumatoid drugs (disease-modifying drugs), such as sulphasalazine, are used to slow disease progression. They require 4–6 months to produce a full response.

Mechanism of action: Sulphasalazine is a combination of salicylate (related to aspirin) and the sulphonamide, sulphapyridine. It may take 6 weeks to produce any therapeutic response. Its mechanism of action is uncertain; it may scavenge the destructive oxygen free radicals which are produced at sites of inflammation, or prevent antigens being absorbed from the colon. Other disease-modifying antirheumatoid drugs are also thought to modify the inflammatory response through various, poorly understood mechanisms.

Pharmacokinetics: Enteric-coated tablets help prevent GI side-effects. Sulphasalazine is metabolised to its components (salicylate and sulphapyridine); which of these is the active ingredient is uncertain.

Side-effects: Sulphasalazine causes nausea, abdominal pains and headache. Skin rashes are common and sulphasalazine should not be used in those allergic to sulphonamides. Bone marrow depression and hepatitis are serious side-effects. Many antirheumatoid drugs produce renal and bone marrow impairment and therefore require regular blood and urine testing. Less severe side-effects are also very common. Hence many patients cannot tolerate these drugs.

Sulphasalazine is also used to treat inflammatory bowel disease.

Other disease-modifying antirheumatoid drugs

Drug	Proposed mechanisms	Adverse effects/comments
Antimalarials (chloroquine)	Inhibit proliferation and activity of immune cells. Stabilise lysosomes and scavenge free radicals	Retinopathy
Penicillamine	Stabilises lysosomes and prevent lymphocyte activation. Inhibit disulphide bridge formation	Metallic taste, nausea, rashes, bone marrow damage, renal damage and oral ulcers
Gold (oral or injections)	Inhibit proliferation and activity of immune cells	Rashes, renal damage, blood disorders and oral ulcers
Cytotoxics (azathioprine, methotrexate)	Prevent DNA synthesis	See Ch. 48. Effective and few side-effects. Good compliance

FIG. 42.1 Complications of rheumatoid arthritis

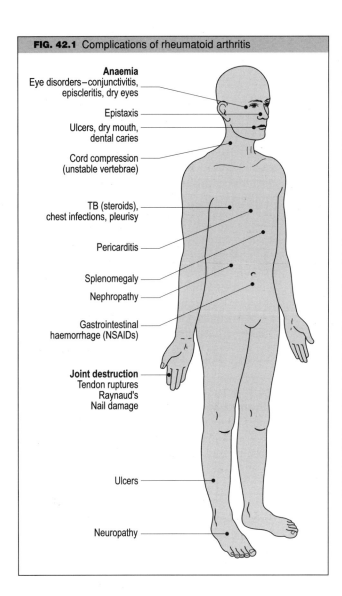

Anaemia
Eye disorders—conjunctivitis, episcleritis, dry eyes

Epistaxis

Ulcers, dry mouth, dental caries

Cord compression (unstable vertebrae)

TB (steroids), chest infections, pleurisy

Pericarditis

Splenomegaly

Nephropathy

Gastrointestinal haemorrhage (NSAIDs)

Joint destruction
Tendon ruptures
Raynaud's
Nail damage

Ulcers

Neuropathy

Progressive stages in the management of rheumatoid arthritis

1. Diagnosis. Exercise to maintain full joint movements.
2. Symptomatic relief with NSAIDs, corticosteroid joint injections and rest in hospital.
3. Prolonged specific antirheumatoid drugs to prevent disease progression.
4. Monitoring and management of complications.
5. Rehabilitation for disabled patients.

REVISION AID
Drugs used in rheumatoid arthritis

- Rheumatoid arthritis is a chronic inflammatory disorder causing joint destruction and many systemic complications

- NSAIDs are used, often with antiulcer drugs, to relieve joint pains

- Exacerbations can be treated with corticosteroid joint injection

- Disease-modifying antirheumatoid drugs, such as sulphasalazine, alter immune responses and slow disease progression. They have a slow onset of action (several months)

- Side-effects of disease-modifying antirheumatoid drugs include GI disturbances, and bone marrow and renal damage. The drugs are often poorly tolerated

43

Drugs and the skin

Eczema

Eczema (or dermatitis) is a skin disorder characterised by an itching, inflammatory rash. Acute eczema presents with a blistered, oozing, oedematous rash while in chronic cases the rash becomes scaled. Eczematous rashes may spread but do not cause scarring. Exogenous or contact eczema occurs in response to an identifiable irritant (e.g. a detergent) or allergen (e.g. zinc). This is treated by avoidance of the precipitating factor. There are numerous forms of endogenous or constitutional eczema. For example, atopic eczema is a genetically determined state related to immunological abnormalities associated with asthma and hay fever. This may arise from a defect of T helper cells.

A dry eczematous rash may be treated with moisturising creams (emollients). A wet rash may be treated with drying solutions (astringents) such as potassium permanganate. These precipitate proteins and reduce serous oozing. They are also antibacterial and reduce secondary infection. Mild topical corticosteroids (e.g. hydrocortisone) can also be used. These are antiinflammatory, immunosuppressive and decrease the rate of epithelial cell proliferation. However systemic absorption can produce numerous, severe side-effects, particularly if very potent corticosteroids are used (see Ch. 41, Glucocorticoids).

Itching may be relieved using antipruritic agents such as calamine, coal tar or sedating antihistamines (H_1-receptor antagonists). Coal tar is a mixture of hydrocarbons which is keratolytic, antiinflammatory and antipruritic. It prevents cellular proliferation by inhibiting DNA synthesis. Unfortunately it is smelly, messy and stains clothing.

Psoriasis

Psoriasis is a chronic skin disease characterised by pink, well-demarcated silvery scaled plaques especially on the extensor surface of the elbows and knees. It affects 2% of adults. Psoriasis is probably an immunological disorder with a genetic predisposition. It may be precipitated by systemic infections, psychological stress, scratching and drugs.

Psoriasis occurs due to excessive epidermal cell proliferation. This may be due to the disturbed function of T cells and immunoglobulins with the abnormal production of inflammatory mediators like leukotrienes, eicosanoids or polyamines (which regulate epidermal proliferation).

Treatment may only be necessary during exacerbations. Keratolytics (e.g. salicylic acid and coal tar) break down keratin causing desquamation and improved penetration of other treatments. Other agents specifically interfere with immune functions (e.g. coal tar and vitamin A derivatives) or nonspecifically inhibit cell division (e.g. cytotoxics).

Sunlight is beneficial in psoriasis possibly by enhancing vitamin D production. Calcipotriol is a topical vitamin D derivative which is odourless and colourless. Hence it is popular with patients and has few side-effects unlike many other psoriasis drugs.

Acne

Acne vulgaris occurs due to blockage of the sebaceous ducts particularly in the face producing spots (papules) which may become inflamed (pustules) due to bacterial digestion of their contents. This arises from a hereditary response to androgenic hormones. Treatment may involve keratolytic/antibacterial washes, prolonged oral antibiotics (e.g. erythromycin), oral contraceptives or, in severe cases, vitamin A derivatives.

Formulations used in dermatology (bases)

- Ointments are greases
- Creams contain emulsions of water and grease which are absorbed more rapidly than ointments
- Pastes consist of a powder mixed into an ointment
- Lotions are liquids of any kind which are less messy on hairy or wet areas

Drugs used in eczema and psoriasis

Drug	Mechanism of action	Notes
Salicylic acid paste	Antiinflammatory and keratolytic	Related to aspirin
Coal tar	Inhibits DNA synthesis	Antiinflammatory, keratolytic and antipruritic Messy and smells
Zinc oxide	Astringent	

Drugs used in eczema

Drug	Mechanism of action	Notes
Topical steroids (e.g. hydrocortisone)	Antiinflammatory and immunosuppressive action	Thins and discolours skin Aggravates infections May cause rebound exacerbation Systemic side-effects
Immunosuppressives (e.g. cyclosporin)	Inhibits interleukin-2 synthesis by T cells	Specialist use only Also used for organ transplants
Calamine lotion	Antipruritic	

Drugs used in psoriasis

Drug	Mechanism of action	Notes
Calcipotriol (topical vitamin D)	Uncertain; reduces epidermal cell proliferation	Avoid in disorders of calcium metabolism
Dithranol	Inhibits DNA synthesis	Stains and irritates skin, so apply only to psoriatic patches
Oral treatment (specialists only)		
Psoralens and UV$_A$ treatment (PUVA)	UV activated psoralens bind DNA and inhibit cell division	May cause skin cancer
Vitamin A derivatives (also used in severe acne)	Antimitotic and immunosuppressive; keratolytic; reduce sebum production	Teratogenic, hepatic and renal damage Also used in severe acne
Immunosuppressives, e.g. methotrexate	Prevents DNA synthesis	See Ch. 48

Glaucoma and mydriatics: timolol and atropine

The aqueous humour is secreted from secretory cells lining the ciliary body. It circulates through the pupil and drains into the trabecular meshwork in the canal of Schlemm. This is located in the angle of the anterior chamber, i.e. between the iris and the conjunctiva (see Fig. 44.1).

Adrenaline and noradrenaline cause dilation of the pupil (mydriasis) and inhibit formation of the aqueous humour. Acetylcholine from parasympathetic neurons causes constriction of the pupil (miosis).

In ophthalmology drugs are often given as eye drops to minimise their systemic effects.

Glaucoma

This is an eye disorder characterised by raised intraocular pressure (above 22 mmHg). This restricts the entry of blood into the eye causing ischaemia of the retina and blindness. Chronic simple glaucoma (the commonest type) is a painless, progressive disorder of older people. The outflow of aqueous humour via the trabecular meshwork is impaired. The exact aetiology is unknown.

Glaucoma is treated with various topical and systemic drugs including β-blockers and parasympathomimetics.

β-Blockers; timolol

Mechanism of action: β-Blockers reduce the secretion of aqueous humour by a direct action on β-receptors of the secretory cells lining the ciliary body.

Side-effects: Topical or systemic β-blockers should not be used in asthma, chronic bronchitis or heart failure as they can aggravate these conditions.

Parasympathomimetic drugs: pilocarpine

Mechanism of action: Pilocarpine is a muscarinic agonist which acts on the intraocular muscles to produce constriction of the pupil. This relieves the crowding around the angle of the anterior chamber, thereby exposing the trabecular meshwork and facilitating drainage of the aqueous humour.

Side-effects: Pilocarpine eye drops produce headaches, dimming and blurring of vision and systemic antimuscarinic side-effects. Unlike β-blockers they can be used for asthmatics.

Acetylcholinesterase inhibitors: These also have a parasympathomimetic effect, by preventing breakdown of acetylcholine. However, today they are rarely used for glaucoma.

Mydriatics/cycloplegics: atropine

Atropine dilates the pupils (mydriasis) and paralyses the ciliary muscles (cycloplegia). This facilitates examination and surgery of the eye.

Mechanism of action: Acetylcholine from parasympathetic terminals causes pupil constriction. All mydriatic/cycloplegic drugs are muscarinic antagonists.

Pharmacokinetics: Atropine eye drops have a prolonged action (up to 10 days). Cyclopentolate is an alternative mydriatic with a shorter duration of action.

Side-effects: Cycloplegics prevent accommodation and cause blurred vision. There is also a small risk of precipitating acute glaucoma by preventing drainage of the aqueous humour. This produces a painful, watering, red eye which must be urgently treated by an ophthalmologist. Systemic antimuscarinic drugs are very unlikely to produce acute glaucoma.

New strategies for the treatment of glaucoma

1. Apraclonidine (an α_2-adrenoceptor agonist) reduces aqueous humour production.

2. Dorzolamide (a topical carbonic anhydrase inhibitor) prevents bicarbonate synthesis and aqueous humour secretion.

3. Prostaglandin analogues which reduce aqueous humour production are also being developed.

REVISION AID
Glaucoma and mydriatics

- Glaucoma is an eye disorder characterised by raised intraocular pressure typically due to impaired drainage of the aqueous humour. This restricts the entry of blood into the eye and ultimately causes blindness

- Chronic simple glaucoma is treated with β-blockers, such as timolol, and with muscarinic agonists (parasympathomimetics)

- β-Blockers reduce the secretion of aqueous humour by a direct action on β-receptors of the secretory cells lining the ciliary body

- The systemic absorption of β-blockers from eye drops can aggravate asthma, chronic bronchitis and heart failure

- Muscarinic antagonists, like atropine, dilate the pupils (mydriasis) and paralyse the ciliary muscles (cycloplegia). This facilitates examination and surgery of the eye

- Antimuscarinic eye drops occasionally precipitate acute glaucoma (a painful, watering red eye) which must be urgently treated by an ophthalmologist

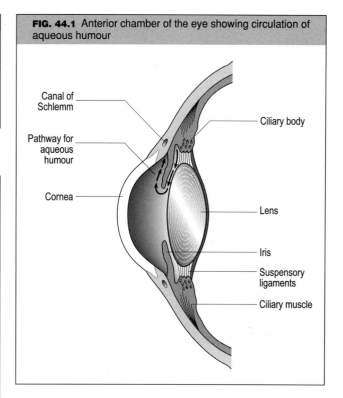

FIG. 44.1 Anterior chamber of the eye showing circulation of aqueous humour

Canal of Schlemm

Pathway for aqueous humour

Cornea

Ciliary body

Lens

Iris

Suspensory ligaments

Ciliary muscle

45 Anticoagulants: heparin and warfarin

Heparin and warfarin are anticoagulants: they prevent the formation of fibrin blood clots (thromboses). Heparin must be used parenterally while warfarin is used orally.

Thromboses typically form in leg veins and break off to lodge in the pulmonary circulation (a pulmonary embolism). This is potentially fatal. Anticoagulants are used in patients with a high risk of thromboembolisms arising from cardiac arrhythmias or valvular heart disease, immobility following trauma or surgery or a past history of thrombosis. They are also used to treat established thrombosis.

Anticoagulation is usually initiated using loading doses of warfarin and heparin with daily monitoring of coagulation times. Guidelines are presented in medical textbooks. See also the table 'Contraindications for anticoagulation'.

Heparin

Heparin is widely used to prevent postoperative thromboses or to produce rapid anticoagulation until warfarin becomes effective.

Mechanism of action: Heparin is a mixture of acidic polysaccharides which are naturally secreted by the liver. Heparin potentiates antithrombin III which inhibits the functioning of six protease enzymes in the coagulation cascade (factors 12a, 11a, 10a, 9, 7a and thrombin; Fig. 45.1). Antithrombin III forms an irreversible complex with these factors, thereby preventing clot formation.

Pharmacokinetics: Heparin cannot be absorbed from the intestines and is used by intravenous or subcutaneous routes to produce rapid anticoagulation. It is inactivated by the liver and has an effective half-life of ~1 hour.

Side-effects: Bleeding is the main complication of heparin. This is treated by stopping further administration. The dose is adjusted by measuring the activated partial thromboplastin time (an assay of the intrinsic coagulation pathway). Rarely, heparin must be neutralised using a strongly basic protein (protamine). Other side-effects include osteoporosis and platelet dysfunction. New low molecular weight heparins are more expensive but may have a lower risk of bleeding.

Oral anticoagulants: warfarin

Mechanism of action: Warfarin blocks the action of vitamin K by competitively inhibiting vitamin K epoxide reductase. This prevents the synthesis in the liver of functional coagulation factors 12, 11, 10, 9 and 7 by preventing posttranslational γ carboxylation of glutamate residues. These residues are important for calcium binding.

Pharmacokinetics: Warfarin is orally active but requires 48–72 hours to produce effective anticoagulation. It has a prolonged effect (4–5 days). Of the drug, 97% is bound to plasma albumin; the remaining free drug enters liver cells to exert its action and undergo metabolism. Warfarin metabolites are excreted in the bile.

Anticoagulation using warfarin is particularly prone to disturbance following interactions with other drugs (see the table 'Factors which disturb anticoagulation with warfarin').

Side-effects: Bleeding is the main complication of warfarin treatment. This may require cessation of therapy and fresh frozen plasma infusions. Vitamin K_1 is a specific antidote but results in resistance to warfarin anticoagulation for 2–3 weeks. The dose of warfarin is adjusted by measuring the prothrombin time or 'INR' International Normalised Ratio (an assay of the extrinsic coagulation pathway).

Warfarin is teratogenic.

Contraindications for anticoagulation

- Severe hypertension
- Recent cerebral haemorrhage
- Peptic ulceration
- Severe liver and renal disease
- Preexisting bleeding disorders
- Major trauma
- Recent surgery, especially to the eye or nervous system
- Hypersensitivity to anticoagulant drugs
- Warfarin is teratogenic and is not used in pregnancy

Factors which disturb anticoagulation with warfarin

Factors which lead to an increased anticoagulant effect and may cause serious bleeding:

- Inhibition of *absorption* of warfarin or vitamin K, e.g. antibiotics, cholestyramine
- Protein-binding *displacement* by drugs, e.g. sulphonamides
- Inhibition of *metabolism*, e.g. by cimetidine, metronidazole
- Potentiation of pharmacological effects, e.g. aspirin inhibits platelet function and also causes bleeding from gastric ulcers
- Disease states which affect drug metabolism or coagulation, e.g. alcoholism, liver and renal disease, hyperthyroidism and heart failure
- Drugs which enhance hepatic metabolism, e.g. antiepileptics

Comparison of anticoagulants

Feature	Heparin	Warfarin
Route	Parenteral	Oral
Mechanism of action	Activates antithombin III	Inhibits synthesis of clotting factors 12, 11, 10, 9, 7 and thrombin
Speed of onset	Immediate	1–3 days
Monitoring	Activated partial thromboplastin time	Prothrombin time (INR)
Duration of effect following cessation of drug	3–6 hours	4–5 days
Specific antidote	Protamine sulphate	Vitamin K
Use in pregnancy	Useful: does not cross placenta	Contraindicated: transplacental and teratogenic

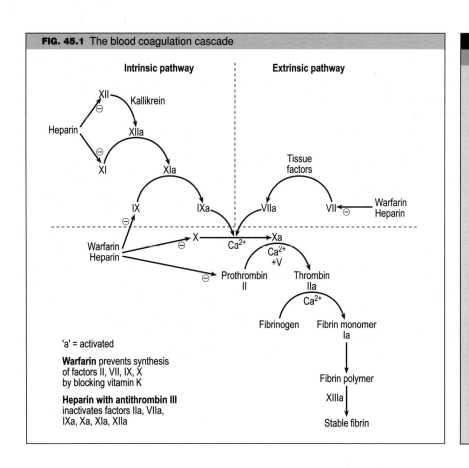

FIG. 45.1 The blood coagulation cascade

'a' = activated

Warfarin prevents synthesis of factors II, VII, IX, X by blocking vitamin K

Heparin with antithrombin III inactivates factors IIa, VIIa, IXa, Xa, XIa, XIIa

46 Antibiotics 1: ampicillin

This chapter, Antibiotics 1, explains the basic principles of antibiotic therapy using the penicillins as examples. The following chapter, Antibiotics 2, illustrates the pharmacology of some other widely used antibiotic agents.

The ideal antibiotic is toxic to microorganisms at concentrations which have little effect on mammalian cells, i.e. it has selective toxicity. Although antibacterial agents are very selective, many other antimicrobial agents produce toxicity in mammalian tissues.

Pharmacokinetics: Antibiotics are usually given orally although there are many routes of administration. Life-threatening infections, particularly meningitis and pneumonia, may require intravenous antibiotic administration. To prevent recurrences, full courses of antibiotics must be completed even when an infection has apparently resolved.

Most antibiotics are excreted by the kidneys.

Side-effects: Allergic rashes are common following administration of many classes of antibiotics. Severe allergic reactions (anaphylaxis) can occur, particularly after injections. Anaphylaxis causes life-threatening hypotension and bronchospasm. Oxygen and adrenaline must be administered urgently.

Diarrhoea commonly occurs because antibiotics kill the normal gut bacteria, leading to colonisation with pathogenic strains. Similarly colonisation by *Candida albicans* (a fungus) causes vaginal thrush.

Resistance: Prolonged or unnecessary use of antibiotics promotes the generation of resistant organisms. Resistance can be minimised by selecting antibiotics according to assays of the bacterial sensitivity.

Mechanisms of antibiotic resistance include: enzymatic inactivation of the drug, expression of resistant forms of the target enzyme, reduction in cellular permeability and expression of an extrusion system (see the table 'Some uses of antibiotics, and mechanisms of resistance').

Inhibitors of cell wall synthesis: ampicillin

Mechanism of action: Ampicillin is a penicillin which is widely used to treat respiratory tract infections (e.g. chronic bronchitis), urinary tract infections (UTIs) and gonorrhoea. Bacterial cell walls consist of alternating units of N-acetylmuramic acid and N-acetylglucosamine. Cytosolic enzymes synthesise these precursors. Cell wall synthesis is completed on the outer surface of the membrane by transpeptidase enzymes which cross-link the polymers. β-Lactam antibiotics (penicillins and cephalosporins) irreversibly inhibit transpeptidases by covalent modification. This prevents cell wall synthesis causing bacteria to lose their shape, lyse and die.

Pharmacokinetics: Probenecid prevents renal elimination of β-lactams and prolongs their action. Ampicillin is poorly absorbed when given orally, and chemical derivatives, such as amoxycillin, are often preferred.

Side-effects: Ampicillin and amoxycillin can cause a rash in patients suffering from glandular fever (which often presents with a sore throat). This rash is often mistaken for an allergic reaction. Of the individuals who develop an allergic reaction to penicillin, 10–15% will react on a subsequent occasion. Of the patients who have an allergic reaction to penicillin, 10% cross-react to cephalosporins.

Penicillins rarely cause encephalopathy.

Some bacteria, especially *Staphylococci*, release β-lactamase enzymes which inactivate β-lactam antibiotics. Hence penicillins may be given with a β-lactamase inhibitor such as clavulanic acid. Some penicillins and cephalosporins (e.g. flucloxacillin and cefuroxime) are less susceptible to β-lactamase and are particularly useful in staphylococcal wound infections, endocarditis and pneumonia.

Some uses of antibiotics, and mechanisms of resistance

Antibiotic	Indications	Mechanism of resistance
Penicillins/cephalosporins	Meningitis, pneumonia, chronic bronchitis, UTI, gonorrhoea	Inactivation by β-lactamase Resistant transpeptidases
Macrolides (erythromycin)	Penicillin allergies, infective diarrhoea, respiratory infections	Resistant ribosomal forms
Aminoglycosides	After urinary and biliary surgery	Enzymatic inactivation by acetylation, adenylylation or phosphorylation
Tetracyclines	*Chlamydia*, chronic bronchitis, acne	Mutation of uptake carrier and enhanced efflux
Chloramphenicol	Bacterial conjunctivitis, meningitis, typhoid	Acetylation by chloramphenicol acetyltransferase
Metronidazole	Anaerobic infections, postoperative prophylaxis	Resistance rare
Quinolones	Gastrointestinal infections, UTIs	Decreased uptake and enhanced efflux
Trimethoprim	Chronic bronchitis, UTIs	Resistant dihydrofolate reductase (DHFR)

FIG. 46.1 Sites of action of some antibiotics

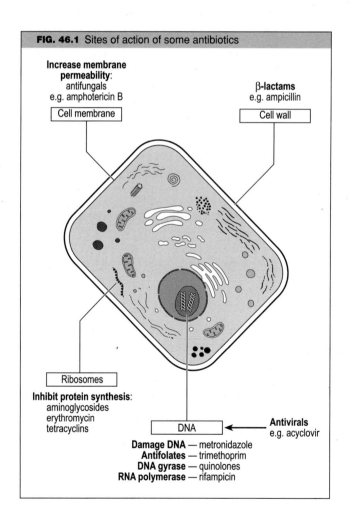

Increase membrane permeability:
antifungals
e.g. amphotericin B

Cell membrane

β-lactams
e.g. ampicillin

Cell wall

Ribosomes

Inhibit protein synthesis:
aminoglycosides
erythromycin
tetracyclins

DNA

Antivirals
e.g. acyclovir

Damage DNA — metronidazole
Antifolates — trimethoprim
DNA gyrase — quinolones
RNA polymerase — rifampicin

47 Antibiotics 2

Protein synthesis inhibitors: erythromycin

1. Macrolides: Erythromycin is an example of this class. Macrolides bind the 50S subunit of bacterial ribosomes, preventing the nascent peptide chain moving through the ribosome. Erythromycin is used as an alternative to penicillin in penicillin-allergic patients, in infective diarrhoeas and respiratory infections. Side-effects include nausea and vomiting.

2. Aminoglycosides: Gentamicin is an aminoglycoside. These prevent initiation of protein synthesis and cause insertion of incorrect amino acids. Bacteria possess an active uptake system for aminoglycosides causing their intracellular accumulation. Gentamicin is used for serious infection, e.g. following urinary or biliary tract surgery. Aminoglycosides cannot be given orally. Side-effects include renal damage, hearing loss and impaired neuromuscular transmission. Plasma level monitoring may be needed.

3. Tetracyclines: Doxycycline is an example of this class. These bind to the 30S subunit of bacterial ribosomes and prevent aminoacyl-tRNA attachment to the A site (where amino acids are added to the nascent peptide). Mammalian ribosomes are also inhibited. However bacteria actively transport tetracyclines into their cytoplasm to generate concentrations 50-fold greater than in mammalian cells. Tetracyclines are used in chlamydial infections, chronic bronchitis and acne. They cause renal damage. They should not be used in children or pregnancy because they stain bones and teeth.

4. Chloramphenicol: This binds to the 50S subunit of bacterial ribosomes near the A site. Chloramphenicol causes irreversible aplastic anaemia and is reserved for life-threatening infections (e.g. meningitis and typhoid) or topical use (e.g. bacterial conjunctivitis). It is particularly active against *Haemophilus influenzae*.

Inhibitors of DNA and RNA synthesis: metronidazole

1. Metronidazole: This is reduced in bacterial cells to unstable metabolites which damage DNA. Metronidazole is particularly active against anaerobic bacteria (which have low redox conditions). It is used in many infections and prophylactically after colonic and gynaecological surgery. Side-effects include gastrointestinal disturbances and unpleasant taste. However resistant organisms rarely develop.

2. Quinolones: Ciprofloxacin is a quinolone. These inhibit DNA gyrase. This prevents supercoiling of bacterial chromosomes and stops DNA replication, expression and repair. Quinolones are used in gastrointestinal and urinary tract infections. They may cause convulsions.

3. Rifampicin: This binds to bacterial RNA polymerase and prevents initiation of transcription. Although resistance develops quickly in many organisms, rifampicin is still used in tuberculosis treatment and prophylaxis. It accelerates the metabolism of many other drugs by inducing liver enzymes.

Folate synthesis inhibitors: trimethoprim
Bacteria cannot take up exogenous folate and must synthesise it from pterdine and p-aminobenzoic acid using dihydropteroate synthetase. This enzyme is inhibited by sulphonamides, such as sulphamethoxazole. Sulphonamides cause a severe skin reaction (Stevens–Johnson syndrome), renal damage, folate deficiency and bone marrow depression. The antiinflammatory drug, sulphasalazine, contains sulphapyridine.

Dihydrofolate reductase (DHFR) converts dihydrofolate to tetrahydrofolate which is essential for synthesis of adenine, guanine, thymidine and methionine. Trimethoprim selectively inhibits bacterial DHFR and ultimately prevents bacterial nucleic acid and protein synthesis. It is used in chronic bronchitis and UTIs.

Sulphamethoxazole and trimethoprim are combined in co-trimoxazole although trimethoprim alone is usually preferred. Folate antagonists may be teratogenic.

Gram negative and Gram positive

Many organisms are classified as to whether or not they stain with Gram's stain. Gram positive organisms have a simpler cell wall, which favours penetration by positively charged molecules, e.g. streptomycin. Gram negative organisms have a more complicated cell wall. Some antibiotics have problems crossing this wall and so are less effective against these gram negative organisms. Such antibiotics include penicillin G, rifampicin and the macrolides.

- Gram positive organisms include: *Staphylococcus* (infections of wounds), *Pneumococcus* (pneumonia) and *Clostridium* (tetanus).

- Gram negative organisms include: *Neisseria meningitis* (meningitis), *Helicobacter pylori* (peptic ulcer) and *Escherichia coli* (urinary infections) – commonly shortened to E. Coli.

REVISION AID
Antibiotics

- Prolonged or unnecessary use of of antibiotics promotes the generation of resistant organisms

- β-Lactam antibiotics (penicillins and cephalosporins) irreversibly inhibit transpeptidases which synthesise bacterial cell walls

- Bacterial protein synthesis is inhibited by macrolides (such as erythromycin), aminoglycosides (such as gentamicin) and tetracyclines (such as doxycycline)

- Metronidazole is reduced in bacterial cells to unstable metabolites which damage DNA. It is particularly active against anaerobic bacteria

- Trimethoprim and sulphonamides prevent bacterial nucleic acid and protein synthesis by inhibiting folate metabolism

- Rarely, severe allergic reactions (anaphylaxis) can cause life-threatening hypotension and bronchospasm. Oxygen and adrenaline must be administered urgently

Other infections and treatments

Tuberculosis: This is a chronic, progressive infection usually affecting the lungs, caused by *Mycobacterium tuberculosis*. Its prevalence worldwide is increasing alarmingly. Management involves 6 months' treatment with isoniazid and rifampicin with the addition of pyrazinamide for the first 2 months. Rifampicin inhibits mycobacterial RNA polymerase. The mechanism of other antitubercular drugs is uncertain.

***Pseudomonas aeruginosa*:** This produces serious infections in burns and wounds and respiratory infections in people with cystic fibrosis. It has a coat which renders it resistant to many antibiotics. Antipseudomonal agents include some penicillins (e.g. piperacillin), aminoglycosides, cefuroximes and quinolones.

Antivirals: These drugs do not eradicate viruses but delay replication. Acyclovir is activated by the viral thymidine kinase present in cells infected with *Herpes simplex*. The metabolite inhibits viral DNA polymerase. Acyclovir is used in shingles, genital herpes, herpes conjunctivitis and encephalitis. It is only active at the start of an infection. Zidovudine (azidothymidine) inhibits retroviral reverse transcriptase. It delays progression of AIDS. It is toxic (particularly to bone marrow).

Antifungals: Clotrimazole is an example of an antifungal. These drugs affect permeability of and transport across fungal cell membranes. They are toxic systemically but are widely used as pessaries against vaginal thrush caused by *Candida albicans*.

Antimalarials: These drugs, of which proguanil is an example, inhibit folate synthesis. The mechanism of action of chloroquine is uncertain.

Insecticides: Insecticides, such as malathion, inhibit acetylcholine esterase. They are used topically against head lice (*Pediculosis humanis capitis*).

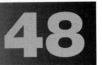

48 Drugs used to treat cancer: cyclophosphamide

Cancer kills one in five people making it the second commonest cause of death. Strictly speaking, 'tumour' is a term for any pathological lump. A malignant tumour (cancer) may metastasise (spread to other organs); a benign tumour cannot.

Symptoms are produced by the physical disruption caused by a tumour (or its metastases), infection of the tumour mass or by-products released from tumour cells (such as hormones). Cytotoxic drugs are used to treat cancer.

Cancer arises due to uncontrolled division of host cells which become invasive, i.e. they can breach epithelial barriers, and metastasise. The aetiology of many forms of cancer is unknown although genome mutations are important factors.

Cytotoxic drugs

The use of cytotoxic drugs alone can only cure 5% of all types of cancer (e.g. leukaemia). Hence they are usually used with radiotherapy and/or surgery. However the prognosis for many common cancers is poor and cytotoxic drugs are used to prolong life rather than cure the disease. Cytotoxics are also used as immunosuppressants in autoimmune conditions such as rheumatoid arthritis.

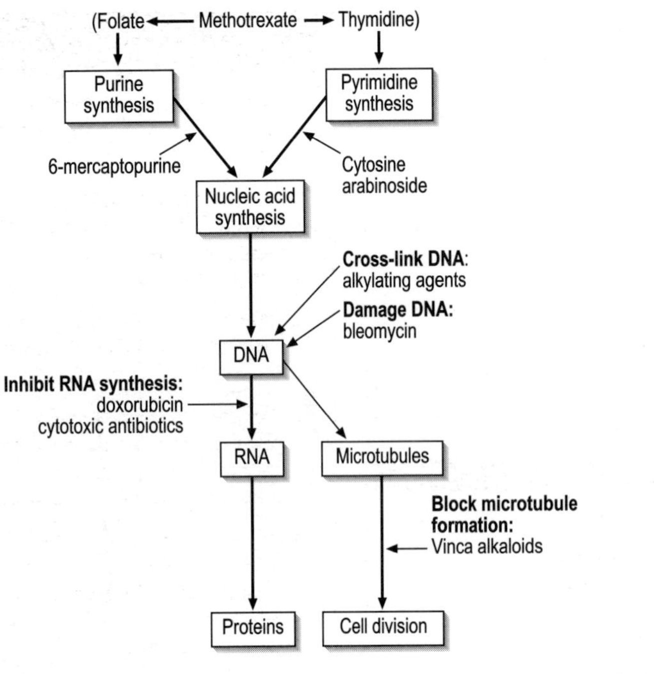

Mechanism of action: Cytotoxic drugs inhibit DNA replication and cell division. They kill a fixed proportion of host and tumour cells (see table 'Drugs used to treat cancer'). Intermittent dosing (e.g. at 3–6 week intervals) is used to deplete the population of cancer cells while allowing a time interval for the recovery of normal tissues. Fortunately normal tissues recover more rapidly than cancer cells. Cytotoxic drugs are often used in combinations to maximise their effectiveness and prevent resistant tumour cells evolving. However this produces more side-effects. Toxicity is greater in rapidly dividing tumour and host cells (e.g. intestine and blood precursors) and many side-effects are due to the toxic action in these tissues.

Pharmacokinetics: Cytotoxic drugs may be administered orally, parenterally or by special routes, e.g. by bladder instillation or intrathecally (into the CSF). Cytotoxic drugs are unusually toxic and special precautions are required to reconstitute them.

Side-effects: See the table 'Common side-effects of cytotoxic drugs'. These represent a major problem, especially bone marrow suppression, which may limit the duration of treatment. Individual agents produce additional side-effects. Cyclophosphamide occasionally produces haemorrhagic cystitis due to accumulation of a metabolite, acrolein, in the bladder. This can be prevented by co-administration of mesna, an antitoxin which is excreted renally.

Biological therapy

This involves the use of naturally occurring compounds which can be used either to suppress the growth of tumour cells or facilitate recovery of host cell population. They include lymphokines (interferons and colony-stimulating factor), growth factors and monoclonal antibodies.

Endocrine therapy: The growth of some tumours, e.g. breast, prostate and endometrial cancers, can be arrested temporarily by hormonal manipulation. This adjuvant therapy may delay the progression of cancer for years.

Oestrogens are used in prostate and breast cancer. The oestrogen antagonist, tamoxifen, is used in breast cancer. Agents that interfere with the synthesis or action of oestrogens or androgen avoid the need for removal of the ovaries or testes in patients with these hormone-sensitive tumours.

FIG. 48.1 Mechanisms of action of cytotoxics

(Folate ◄—— Methotrexate ——► Thymidine)

Purine synthesis → Pyrimidine synthesis

6-mercaptopurine → Nucleic acid synthesis ← Cytosine arabinoside

Nucleic acid synthesis →

Cross-link DNA: alkylating agents

Damage DNA: bleomycin

DNA

Inhibit RNA synthesis: doxorubicin cytotoxic antibiotics →

RNA → Microtubules

Block microtubule formation: ◄—— Vinca alkaloids

Proteins → Cell division

Drugs used to treat cancer

Drug	Mechanism of action	Uses	Specific side-effects
Alkylating agents: **Cyclophosphamide**	Covalently cross-links DNA strands	Leukaemia, lymphoma, solid tumours	Infertility, leukaemia, haemorrhagic cystitis
Platinum analogues: **Cisplatin**	Covalently cross-links DNA strands	Ovarian and testicular cancer	Nephrotoxic, neuropathies, deafness
Cytotoxic antibiotics: **Doxorubicin**	Intercalates between DNA nucleotides	Leukaemia, lymphoma, solid tumours	Enhances radiotoxicity, cardiotoxic
Bleomycin	Damages DNA		Less toxic to bone marrow but causes pulmonary fibrosis
Antimetabolites: **Methotrexate**	Prevents nucleic acid synthesis, e.g. by inhibiting folate synthesis	Intrathecally for CNS tumours and nonmalignant disease	Renal elimination; accumulates in extracellular fluid causing pneumonitis
Cytosine arabinoside	Inhibits pyrimidine synthesis	Leukaemia	
6-Mercaptopurine	Inhibits purine synthesis	Leukaemia	
Vinca alkaloids: **Vincristine**	Prevents microtubule formation	Leukaemia, lymphoma, solid tumours	Neuropathies Less bone marrow toxicity
Antioestrogen: **Tamoxifen**	Oestrogen receptor antagonist	Breast cancer	Hypercalcaemia (rare)
Antiandrogen: **Goserelin**	LHRH analogue, reduces testosterone levels	Prostate cancer	Transient increase in tumour activity

---

FIG. 48.2 Side-effects of cytotoxics

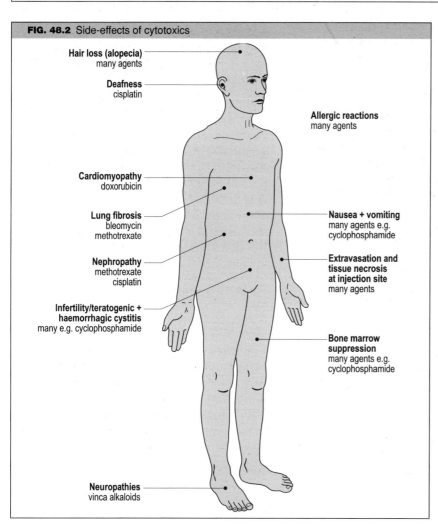

Hair loss (alopecia)
many agents

Deafness
cisplatin

Cardiomyopathy
doxorubicin

Lung fibrosis
bleomycin
methotrexate

Nephropathy
methotrexate
cisplatin

Infertility/teratogenic +
haemorrhagic cystitis
many e.g. cyclophosphamide

Neuropathies
vinca alkaloids

Allergic reactions
many agents

Nausea + vomiting
many agents e.g.
cyclophosphamide

Extravasation and
tissue necrosis
at injection site
many agents

Bone marrow
suppression
many agents e.g.
cyclophosphamide

Immunosuppressants

These are used to prevent rejection of transplanted organs and in the specialist management of autoimmune diseases such as psoriasis and rheumatoid arthritis. They produce bone marrow suppression and make patients prone to infection. Azathioprine is metabolised into the purine analogue, 6-mercaptopurine, which inhibits DNA synthesis and cell division. Side-effects are similar to other cytotoxic drugs. Cyclosporin has little myelotoxic effect but causes renal damage. It prevents proliferation of T cells, possibly by blocking the activity of interleukin-2.

Glucocorticoids (e.g. prednisolone): These are widely used as immunosuppressives and also prevent the growth of many tumours (see Ch. 41, Glucocorticoids).

REVISION AID
Drugs used to treat cancer

- Cytotoxic drugs are used in combinations to cure or palliate cancer

- Cytotoxic drugs prevent cell division in host and tumour cells; however host cells recover more quickly than tumour cells

- They are administered at monthly intervals so that host tissues can recover

- Cytotoxic drugs have many serious side-effects particularly affecting blood precursors, the intestines or reproductive system

- Naturally occurring compounds such as hormones, hormone antagonists and growth factors are used as adjuvants to other cancer treatment

Common side-effects of cytotoxic drugs

1. Bone marrow suppression causing anaemia, bleeding disorders and immunosuppression; regular blood tests required
2. Nausea and vomiting; may be prevented by antiemetic premedication
3. Extravasation at the site of injection; may cause severe tissue damage
4. Reversible hair loss (alopecia)
5. Teratogenic; contraception advisable
6. Male sterility; may necessitate sperm storage

49 Side-effects

Side-effects (toxic effects or adverse reactions) refer to the unwanted effects of a drug. All drugs produce side-effects. Figure 49.1 gives some examples. Of hospital patients, 10–20% suffer drug side-effects.

Some drugs produce serious side-effects at, or near therapeutic concentrations, which may limit or prevent further treatment. These are said to have a low toxic:therapeutic index. They include: warfarin (causes bleeding); lithium (renal and CNS damage); gentamicin (renal damage); digoxin (arrhythmias); insulin (hypoglycaemia), and cytotoxic drugs (bone marrow depression, nausea and vomiting). Chronically administered systemic corticosteroids also produce many side-effects.

Therapeutic monitoring: Measurements of plasma drug concentrations (or biological assays) can be used to identify toxicity. Therapeutic drug monitoring is also required: to guide further treatment, e.g. following paracetamol or aspirin overdose, to monitor patient compliance, and to check that an effective plasma concentration is being achieved (e.g. with antiepileptics and antibiotics). Plasma drug levels are determined routinely during the use of digoxin, lithium, gentamicin and methylxanthines.

Antimuscarinic side-effects: Many antipsychotics, antidepressants, antiemetics and H_1-receptor antagonists (antihistamines) produce side-effects by acting as antagonists at muscarinic receptors. These anticholinergic side-effects include dry mouth, blurred vision, urinary retention, constipation and confusion.

Allergic reactions: There is a danger of severe anaphylactic reaction following the administration of a drug to which a patient is allergic. Hence development of an allergic reaction (such as a rash) precludes future use of that agent. Antibiotics cause many allergic drug reactions, partly because they are widely prescribed. Streptokinase is particularly allergenic and is contraindicated between 5 days and 1 year of a previous exposure. Allergic reactions are not dose-dependent

side-effects. They are examples of idiosyncratic or unpredictable side-effects which are unrelated to the main actions of a drug.

Teratogens: A teratogen is an agent which causes physical defects in the developing embryo. Drugs are generally avoided during pregnancy or in women who intend to become pregnant. When the use of drugs is unavoidable, older agents which are known to be safe are often used (e.g. α-methyldopa for hypertension or promethazine for severe vomiting).

Relatively few drugs are known to be human teratogens although some examples include alcohol, anticonvulsants, warfarin, lithium and cytotoxics.

Side-effects and drug development: Drug development involves discovery of a suitable compound (based on rational design or serendipity) and extensive pharmacological and toxicity testing in animals. A Clinical Trial Certificate may then be obtained from the Committee on Safety of Medicines (CSM). Phase I trials are then conducted to obtain pharmacological, pharmacokinetic and safety data in 25–50 healthy volunteers. Phase II trials allow dose-finding, efficacy and further safety studies in 50–100 patients. Phase III trials are full clinical trials designed to test efficacy and identify side-effects in 250–1000 patients.

Because pre-marketing trials rarely involve more than 2000 subjects, they will only identify common side-effects (i.e. side-effects affecting more than 1 patient in 750). Less frequent side-effects are detected by postmarketing surveillance, either by formal (Phase IV) trials or by the voluntary reporting of suspected side-effects by doctors (e.g. using the yellow cards inserted in the British National Formulary). Unfortunately this voluntary reporting to the CSM has a low response rate.

Side-effects which are rare, which resemble a common disease or which imitate the disease under treatment are particularly hard to detect (e.g. anxiety following benzodiazepine withdrawal).

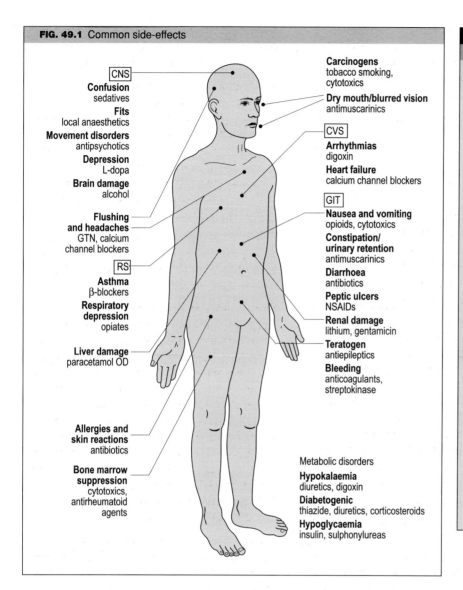

FIG. 49.1 Common side-effects

CNS

Confusion
sedatives

Fits
local anaesthetics

Movement disorders
antipsychotics

Depression
L-dopa

Brain damage
alcohol

**Flushing
and headaches**
GTN, calcium
channel blockers

RS

Asthma
β-blockers

**Respiratory
depression**
opiates

Liver damage
paracetamol OD

**Allergies and
skin reactions**
antibiotics

**Bone marrow
suppression**
cytotoxics,
antirheumatoid
agents

Carcinogens
tobacco smoking,
cytotoxics

Dry mouth/blurred vision
antimuscarinics

CVS

Arrhythmias
digoxin

Heart failure
calcium channel blockers

GIT

Nausea and vomiting
opioids, cytotoxics

**Constipation/
urinary retention**
antimuscarinics

Diarrhoea
antibiotics

Peptic ulcers
NSAIDs

Renal damage
lithium, gentamicin

Teratogen
antiepileptics

Bleeding
anticoagulants,
streptokinase

Metabolic disorders

Hypokalaemia
diuretics, digoxin

Diabetogenic
thiazide, diuretics, corticosteroids

Hypoglycaemia
insulin, sulphonylureas

50 Miscellaneous topics

Gout: allopurinol

Gout is a painful disorder due to urate crystal deposition in joints. It typically affects the big toe. Uric acid, a by-product of nucleic acid metabolism, can achieve high plasma concentrations following increased production (e.g. malignant disease) or reduced excretion. Gout is promoted by diuretics and alcohol excess. Acute attacks are treated with analgesics (e.g. indomethacin). Prophylactic drugs include allopurinol which prevents urate synthesis by inhibiting xanthine oxidase. Probenecid (a uricosuric) competes with the renal urate reabsorption mechanism to promote urate secretion. Allopurinol and uricosurics aggravate acute attacks.

Paracetamol poisoning: acetylcysteine

Paracetamol is the drug most commonly used in deliberate self-poisoning. Overdose overloads the capacity of the liver to detoxify paracetamol by glucuronidation, sulphation or conjugation with glutathione. This causes generation of toxic metabolites and potentially fatal liver damage. Intravenous acetylcysteine increases glutathione formation and protects the liver up to 24 hours after paracetamol ingestion.

Iron and anaemia

Iron deficiency is the commonest cause of anaemia. It produces characteristic hypochromic, microcytic red blood cells usually as a consequence of chronic blood loss (e.g. following heavy periods or gastrointestinal diseases including cancer). Oral iron supplements can correct this and may be given prophylactically in pregnancy. Oral iron may cause nausea, constipation or diarrhoea and abdominal pains.

Iron overload can occur following accidental poisoning, particularly in children, or following repeated blood transfusions (e.g. in thalassaemias). Chelating agents, such as desferrioxamine, are administered to bind the iron and promote its excretion.

Antiemetics: prochlorperazine and metoclopramide

Antiemetics are used for the symptomatic relief of nausea and vomiting (e.g. following administration of opioid analgesics or cytotoxic drugs). Prochlorperazine is a dopamine D_2-receptor antagonist which acts centrally (in the chemoreceptor trigger zone) to prevent nausea. Metoclopramide acts on central and intestinal dopamine receptors. It increases gastric emptying and is therefore avoided in intestinal obstruction. Both these agents can produce acute movement disorders, such as oculogyric crises, particularly in young women. (These attacks can be treated with muscarinic antagonists.)

Other antiemetic drugs include histamine H_1-receptor antagonists, cannabinoids, muscarinic and $5-HT_3$-receptor antagonists.

Sedation is a common side-effect of antiemetics.

H_1-receptor antagonists: terfenadine

H_1-receptor antagonists (antihistamines) are used as antiemetics (e.g. in motion sickness), as antipruritics to relieve itching, as sedatives in many proprietary cold cures and in the treatment of allergic reaction and vertigo. The older agents, such as chlorpheniramine, are more sedating and may act as antagonists at dopamine, 5-HT, α_1-adrenergic and muscarinic receptors with consequent side-effects.

Newer, more selective agents, such as terfenadine, are less sedating and are used to treat allergic conditions including hay fever. However H_1-receptor antagonists have little in common with the H_2-receptor antagonists used in peptic ulcer disease.

Drugs used in obstetrics: oxytocin

Prostaglandins E and F, ergometrine (an ergot alkaloid) and oxytocin are used to induce abortions, induce or augment labour and to minimise the blood loss from the placental site following delivery, miscarriage or abortion. Oxytocin is a naturally occurring hormone which can be infused or injected. It produces regular coordinated contractions of the uterus which assists labour. However its effects may not be potent enough to initiate labour or treat severe postpartum haemorrhage. Consequently prostaglandins may be required, although these cause gastrointestinal disturbances. Ergotamine is a partial agonist of α_1 and 5-HT$_1$ receptors. It causes peripheral vasoconstriction and hypertension. Large doses of oxytocin, or related agents, may produce sustained uterine contractions and foetal death.

Clomiphene and infertility

Clomiphene is an antioestrogen which inhibits the normal negative feedback of oestrogens on the hypothalamus and pituitary. This leads to increased secretion of gonadotrophins which stimulate the ovaries. Five-day courses may be given at the start of the menstrual cycle to enhance ovulation. This is used to treat infertility due to lack of ovulation. Clomiphene may cause multiple pregnancies.

Myaesthenia gravis: pyridostigmine

Myaesthenia gravis is a rare condition in which antibodies attack nicotinic receptors on skeletal muscle. This causes muscular weakness and paralysis. It is treated with acetylcholinesterase inhibitors such as pyridostigmine. These prevent acetylcholine breakdown and prolong its action in the neuromuscular cleft. This allows acetylcholine to reach the few remaining receptors on the skeletal muscle membrane.

Excessive use of acetylcholinesterase inhibitors will aggravate muscular weakness because excess acetylcholine produces a depolarising blockade. This is termed a cholinergic crisis.

Shorter acting acetylcholinesterase inhibitors, such as edrophonium, are used to diagnose myaesthenia gravis: a single test-dose will usually improve muscle strength in myaesthenics. Edrophonium will also improve muscle strength in patients receiving inadequate acetylcholinesterase inhibitors. However if patients are receiving excessive acetylcholinesterase inhibitors, edrophonium will either have no effect or aggravate weakness.

Appendix 1: Quantitative aspects of receptor theory

It is possible to measure the number of receptors occupied by a drug. This involves the use of a drug (or radioligand) which is radioactive and is selective for particular receptors. In these radioligand binding experiments, tissues are exposed to small amounts of radioactive drug which compete with known concentrations of unlabelled drug for binding sites on the receptor. The radioactivity in the tissue will then indicate the proportion of radioligand which has not been displaced by the unlabelled drug. If the unlabelled drug has a high affinity for the receptors it will occupy a large proportion of them at low concentrations and the tissue will contain little radioactivity. By using several concentrations of unlabelled drugs it is possible to construct a radioligand binding curve. These are sigmoidal curves which show the displacement of radioligand by increasing concentrations of unlabelled drug and allow calculation of the Kd and Hill slope. The dissociation constant, Kd, is the concentration of a drug required to occupy half of the available receptors. The dissociation constant is an estimate of affinity (not efficacy) and is calculated in the same manner for agonists and antagonists. The Hill slope coefficient is derived from the gradient of the linear part of the binding curve: a value of 1 indicates no cooperativity, values less than 1 indicate negative cooperativity while values greater than 1 indicate positive cooperativity.

In radioligand binding experiments the amount of radioligand in the tissue is being measured not the tissue's physiological response to the drug. Potency, efficacy and EC50 values refer to concentration–response curves whilst affinity and Kd refer to binding curves.

The *Langmuir equation* is used to calculate the receptor occupancy by a drug. It states:

$$pA = \frac{[x]}{[x] + K_A}$$

where pA is the proportion of receptors occupied by drug x; [x] is the concentration of the drug and K_A is its dissociation constant.

The *Schild equation* is used to predict the response to an antagonist. It states:

$$r = 1 + \frac{[B]}{K_B}$$

where r is the concentration ratio (i.e. the ratio of the concentration of an agonist that produces a specified response in the presence of an antagonist to the agonist concentration that produces the same response in the absence of the antagonist), [B] is the concentration of a competitive antagonist and K_B is its dissociation constant.

Quantification of antagonism It has proven difficult to quantify the responses to antagonists because their responses depend on the agonist used. One attempt is to state the Kd (see above) or pA2 (see under Concentration–Response Curves). Alternatively the concentration ratio may be used (see above). Finally the IC50 can be used. This is the molar concentration of an antagonist that reduces a specified response to 50% of its former value. Unfortunately the IC50 may also indicate the molar concentration of an agonist which reduces a response to 50% of its former value where the response produced is an inhibitory response; or the molar concentration of a drug which displaces 50% of a radioligand from binding sites in a tissue.

Further reading

General textbooks

Aikenhead A R, Smith G 1995 Textbook of anaesthesia, 3rd edn. Churchill Livingstone, Edinburgh

British National Formulary 1996 British Medical Association/Royal Pharmaceutical Society of Great Britain, London

Conway J, Bilski A 1990 β-blockers. In: Ganten D, Mulrow P J (eds) Handbook of experimental pharmacology 93, Springer-Verlag, pp 65–105

Grahame-Smith D G, Aronson J K 1992 Oxford textbook of clinical pharmacology and drug therapy, 2nd edn. Oxford University Press, Oxford

Kazda S, Knott A 1990 Calcium antagonists. In: Ganten D, Mulrow P J (eds) Handbook of experimental pharmacology 93, Springer-Verlag, pp 301–377

Kendell R E, Zealley A K 1993 Companion to psychiatric studies. Churchill Livingstone, Edinburgh

Kramer H J 1990 Diuretics. In: Ganten D, Mulrow P J (eds) Handbook of experimental pharmacology 93, Springer-Verlag, pp 21–65

Kumar P, Clark M 1994 Clinical medicine, 3rd edn. Baillière Tindall, London

Rang H P, Dale M M, Ritter J M 1995 Pharmacology, 3rd edn. Churchill Livingstone, Edinburgh

More specialised references

Chard T, Lilford R 1990 Basic sciences for obstetrics and gynaecology, 3rd edn. Springer-Verlag, London

Franks N P, Lieb W R 1994 Molecular and cellular mechanisms of general anaesthesia. Nature 367:607–614

Hille B 1992 Ionic channels of excitable membranes, 2nd edn. Sinauer Associates, Massachusetts

Hoffbrand A V, Pettit J E 1992 Essential haematology, 3rd edn. Blackwell Scientific, Oxford

Hugo W B, Russel A D 1992 Pharmaceutical microbiology, 5th edn. Blackwell Scientific, Oxford

Hunter J A A, Savin J A, Dahl M V 1995 Clinical dermatology, 2nd edn. Blackwell Scientific, Oxford

Jeffcoate W 1993 Lecture notes in endocrinology, 5th edn. Blackwell Scientific, Oxford

Jenkinson D H et al 1995 IUP recommendations on terms and symbols in quantitative pharmacology. Pharmacological Review 47:255–266

Kruk Z L, Pycock C J 1991 Neurotransmitters and drugs, 3rd edn. Chapman and Hall, London

Opie L H 1991 Drugs for the heart, 3rd edn. W B Saunders, Philadelphia

Porter D R, Sturrock R D 1993 Medical management of rheumatoid arthritis. British Medical Journal 307:425–428

Pratt W B, Taylor P (eds) 1990 Principles of drug action, 3rd edn. Churchill Livingstone, Edinburgh

Royal College of Psychiatrists 1987 Drug scenes. Royal College of Psychiatrists, London

Ruffolo R R 1982 Important concepts of receptor theory. Journal of Autonomic Pharmacology 2:277–295

Sirtoir C R, Manzoni C, Larati M R 1991 Mechanism of lipid-lowering agents. Cardiology 78:226–235

Unger T, Gohlke P, Gruber M G 1990 Converting enzyme inhibitors. In: Ganten D, Mulrow P J (eds) Handbook of experimental pharmacology 93, Springer-Verlag, pp 377–483

Watson S, Girdlestone D 1996 Ion channel and receptor supplement. Trends in Pharmacological Sciences, 6th edn.

INDEX

Note: numbers in bold refer to Figures,
numbers in italics refer to Tables.